Additional Praise for

The Essential Oils
Hormone Solution

"Dr. Mariza is smart, honest, and committed to creating powerful, natural solutions for women who don't want to take synthetic hormones. She pairs the power of plant-based therapy with effective lifestyle habits to move the needle in women's hormone health."

—Kellyann Petrucci, MS, ND, *New York Times* bestselling author of
Dr. Kellyann's Bone Broth Diet and *The 10-Day Belly Slimdown*

"Essential oils have a meaningful impact on your biology. Dr. Mariza Snyder elegantly distills the latest science into an easy-to-read, actionable plan, showing women how to use them in effective ways to take control of everyday hormone issues. Dr. Mariza's protocols are the key to lasting energy and focus."

—Dave Asprey, *New York Times* bestselling author
of *The Bulletproof Diet* and *Head Strong*

"In *The Essential Oils Hormone Solution*, Dr. Mariza Snyder takes the benefits of essential oils to another level by harnessing their plant-based power to achieve balanced hormones without the need for conventional hormone therapy. This is a game changer in women's health and something that anyone dealing with fatigue, weight-loss resistance, stress, or other hormone-related problems needs to read immediately to start feeling the way you are designed to feel—vibrant and thriving."

—Dr. Will Cole, bestselling author of *Ketotarian*

"This book should be on every woman's book shelf. An in-depth exploration of the science of oils in supporting women's health in the most sacred, nurturing, and safe ways."

—Magdalena Wszelaki, bestselling author of *Cooking for Hormone Balance*

"Dr. Mariza has been there herself—she has experienced hormonal turmoil and discovered the power of essential oils to bring her hormones back into balance and reclaim her body. In her book *The Essential Oils Hormone Solution*, she has shortened the learning curve for women who also struggle with hormonal balance and are seeking a natural alternative to heal. The wisdom and knowledge, as well as practical tips, essential oil blend recipes, and a step-by-step program, that she shares in her book is invaluable, especially for those of us who have polycystic ovary syndrome (PCOS)."

—Amy Medling, author of *Healing PCOS* and founder of PCOS Diva

The
Essential Oils
Hormone
Solution

The Essential Oils Hormone Solution

Reclaim Your Energy and Focus and Lose Weight Naturally

Dr. Mariza Snyder

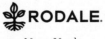 RODALE.

New York

*I dedicate this book to my mom for inspiring me to follow my heart
and passion and for being with me on our hormone journey.*

CONTENTS

Introduction   1

PART I
A HORMONE AND ESSENTIAL OIL PRIMER
13

CHAPTER 1   How to Balance Your Hormones Without Adding Hormones   15

CHAPTER 2   The Guide to Using Essential Oils   37

CHAPTER 3   The Top 15 Essential Oils for Hormones and the Value of Daily Usage   58

CHAPTER 4   The Importance of Creating Your Own Essential-Oil Rituals   64

PART II
USING ESSENTIAL OILS TO ADDRESS YOUR HORMONAL SYMPTOMS
73

CHAPTER 5   Stress   75

CHAPTER 6   Energy and Fatigue   94

CHAPTER 7   Sleep Issues   114

CHAPTER 8   Weight Issues   134

CHAPTER 9   Female Hormones:
Fertility, Perimenopause, and Menopause   151

CHAPTER 10   Libido   169

CHAPTER 11   Emotions: Balancing Anxiety, Depression, and
Mood Swings   186

CHAPTER 12   Cognitive Issues: Memory and Concentration   208

CHAPTER 13   Digestive Issues   227

CHAPTER 14   Toxicity   241

PART III

THE 14-DAY RESCUE PLAN TO JUMP-START YOUR HORMONAL HEALTH

269

CHAPTER 15   The Five Pillars of a Foundational Lifestyle   275

CHAPTER 16   The 14-Day Rescue Meal Plan Basics   306

CHAPTER 17   The 14-Day Rescue Meal Plan and Recipes   313

CHAPTER 18   Refresh and Replenish   345

APPENDIX A   Resources   351

APPENDIX B   Bibliography   355

Acknowledgments   381

Index   385

Introduction

I have a confession to make. Not long ago, I was a health-care practitioner leading a double life. By day, I greeted patients, listened to their concerns, and did my best to find the missing link. But in the midst of it all, I found myself struggling with the same symptoms they suffered from, and I did my best to hide that from the world. I put on my happy mask and pushed forward, ignoring the signs that something was seriously off-balance.

The questions I asked my patients to get to the bottom of their deep-rooted problems were precisely the same questions I should have been asking myself:

Are you gaining weight and don't know why?

Is your energy drained?

Do you have trouble falling asleep and then have to drag yourself out of bed in the morning?

My own answer to every question was "Yes."

Are you craving ice cream or potato chips in the middle of the day and/or late at night?

Do you find your keys in the freezer and your glasses on top of the toilet?

Have you sent the same text to your friend for the third time after forgetting about the previous two?

Sadly, I was preaching to the choir. Every symptom they described, I, too, was experiencing.

Are you so moody that your husband approaches with caution when he sees your face?

Do you often feel like you're just losing your mind?

My patients were continually astounded at my mind-reading superpowers while I fought to swallow that gut feeling that kept creeping back up. Of course, deep down I knew. Looking at their faces was like looking in a mirror. And the culprit?

Hormonal imbalance.

The first step to figuring out answers is realizing that what you are experiencing *isn't normal*. But even though my symptoms paralleled those of my patients, I refused to take my own advice. After all, it's so much easier to ignore what you know you need to do. Chronically fatigued and burnt out, I ran myself into the ground until the stress spun me into a downward spiral of illness. My immune system needed some love, but instead I just ignored my body and my intuition, and I pushed on forward.

I felt like a failure. What kind of doctor can't even heal herself? Outwardly successful but completely lost as to why I was suffering, I continued to allow my double life to grind me down for years. As women, we pride ourselves and develop a sense of self based on how well we can take care of our families, take care of ourselves, and take care of the world, but when you feel like you're failing yourself, how can you begin to empower anyone else?

The tricky thing about hormonal imbalance is that it often sneaks around in the background, wreaking havoc on your health before you even know it's there. As a result, doctors may dismiss your symptoms or attribute them to something else entirely, as mine did, leaving you wondering what is really going on in your body and if you will ever feel great again.

Add to that the environmental factors that played a role in the imbalance; air pollutants, chemicals in food, synthetic estrogens in beauty products, and the constant stress driving our emotional lives are the iceberg lurking beneath the surface. The only thing that doctors see is our list of symptoms and they assume that fluctuating hormones in early life and declining hormonal levels as we age are the culprit of our problems. But they affect women of all ages, even young girls beginning their cycles. Sleep, mood, weight, energy, libido, cravings, and basic functioning—all are at the mercy of our hormones.

What finally pulled me out was discovering the power of high-quality essential oils paired with lifestyle changes. They transformed my life and allowed me to recalibrate my hormonal levels. And they can do the same for you!

I discovered a new sense of empowerment after solving my own hormonal health crisis, and have made it my personal mission to share this with women everywhere. I've spent the last five years devoted to incorporating essential oils into individualized healthcare plans for both my patients and my readers with incredible success, particularly because my focus has been on women's hormone health. Many of these women had given up, assuming that what they were experiencing was their new normal. They resigned themselves to living with suboptimal health, struggling with bodies they no longer recognized.

These women were no different from you and me—they simply wanted effective solutions to their hormonal issues. When I shared with them the power behind essential oils and how they could help to bridge the gap between lifestyle changes and hormonal imbalance, they were thrilled. Regaining vitality, while knowing that they would have an empowering ally in their fight against hormonal chaos, gave them the strength to try one more potential solution to their own hormonal imbalance.

If you've never experienced aromatherapy or the power that a single drop of high-quality essential oil holds, then you may be skeptical. Here's the truth: essential oils are natural aromatic compounds found in the roots, seeds, stems, bark, leaves, and flowers of various plants. They are super-charged, fifty to seventy times more potent than their dried-herbal counterparts. They're simply the best plant-based remedy that exists, and they have been successfully used for thousands of years.

With instantaneous results and the ability to use them as needed, there is virtually no downside to using essential oils when you use them safely. Within minutes you will experience results. Essential oils are a game-changer. Once you begin to experience their power, they will become an important part of your daily routine, empower you to make foundational changes in your health-care regimen, and leave you with increased vitality and a balanced mind and body.

How This Book Came to Be

When I was a child, a serious car accident left me with a concussion and whiplash that led to chronic headaches and migraines. My immune system was so stressed I was constantly ill—colds, the flu, strep throat, sinus infections. Despite these circumstances, I persevered, graduated from college with plans to become a doctor, and began working as a biochemist at the Lawrence Livermore National Laboratory to save up for medical school. Over the years, I continued to suffer from the same symptoms and enlisted the help of countless experts. When nothing they prescribed worked, I tried to accept the fact that living with chronic pain and succumbing to frequent illness just might be my normal. I was even told that my chronic migraine pain was something I was going to deal with for the rest of my life.

Luckily, a co-worker saw through the façade and suggested that I visit a functional medicine practice with a team of functional chiropractors and nutritionists. At this point, I had nothing to lose, so I went—and thank God I did. After only two months of treatment, my migraines slowly dissipated before vanishing entirely. I was in shock!

My entire paradigm shifted. I chucked my medical school plans and went to chiropractic school instead. Empowered to help others the way I had been helped, I devoted my life to a functional, individualistic health-care practice, highly specialized in neurologically driven, upper-cervical-specific, and systemic issues. Many of my patients were women over the age of forty who came in for treatment of migraines, diabetes, insomnia, chronic fatigue, fibromyalgia, insomnia, and what they called "female problems." Mid-thirties to forties is typically when female hormones naturally start to slowly shift and decline, but it is also the age when any bad habits start to catch up with you. Now, add in the unrelenting stress from family commitments, work, finances, and everything else that life throws at you, and you have a whole host of problems on your hands. My patients didn't just have chronic pain and migraines; they also had too much on their plates, which in turn led to zapped energy, sleeplessness, moodiness, headaches, bloating, and weight gain.

Sadly, because their doctors only saw the symptoms and not the whole patient, they were quick to downplay their needs and ignore the root problem. More often than not, the doctors prescribed antidepressants simply because their patients' symptoms pointed to depression and anxiety, but it didn't make these women feel better. This chronic misdiagnosis made me more determined than ever to help them, so I became an expert in nutrition and shifted the focus of my practice.

But, as we often do, I became so driven to help women like myself that I lost sight of my own needs. During my late twenties, when I was getting my doctorate as a practitioner, I overloaded myself and didn't listen to the warning signs. I spiraled downward into a deep illness. I could barely drag myself out of bed in the morning, and fell asleep during classes and when working in the lab. I suffered from what I now know to be hormone-related weight resistance. I became extremely irritable and anxious, and dealt with horrendous monthly periods and mood swings. By my early thirties, not much had changed. I was still moody, irritable, and exhausted owing to the trifecta of adrenal fatigue, estrogen overload, and my family history of hormonal imbalance.

I now recognize that I come from a line of women who've struggled with their hormones, starting with my maternal grandmother. Owing to toxic exposure at her job, my grandma experienced what we now know as estrogen dominance from a bombardment of xenoestrogens, or chemicals that mimic estrogenic effects. My mom, my sister, and I always had problems with our hormones, especially around our menstrual cycle, pointing to estrogen dominance just like my grandmother's. Growing up, I didn't understand why my mom always had unexplained weight gain, cravings, severe mood swings, and, most important, a consistent lack of energy. When puberty rocked my world and I began to experience similar symptoms, we didn't talk about it. As time passed, I didn't deal with it well— I ate the wrong things, drank too much coffee, and never slowed down enough to admit that my overachieving go-go-go lifestyle was making things worse.

The other factor playing a role in my health crisis was my belief in prioritizing my health and self care. Growing up, I believed that my worth as a woman was measured by how much I was able to do for other people. I was determined to prove my worth through hard work, serving others and adding more to my plate. At some point my plate became a massive, unmanageable platter and yet I still found myself stressing about not doing enough, especially for other people. I was convinced that self care was selfish and self-indulgent. I remember calling my workouts at the gym my selfish hour. That was how powerful my disempowering mindset was for most of my life.

During this time, I was not myself anymore; I felt like a robot simply going through the motions—until I took a deep look at the decisions I made about my health, lifestyle, and happiness. I was unhappy and unhealthy. I experienced a lot of shame because I had no energy reserves to show up and serve my patients. Women, like myself, often feel the need to get permission to love ourselves and treat ourselves with respect, but whose permission are we waiting for?

The biggest way we limit ourselves is in how we take care of everyone else first and put ourselves last. And the only way to shift the priority is to shift our belief in how we feel about ourselves. Often our belief is that our worth and value are based on what we do for others. Shifting that belief mindset means we make ourselves the priority, that we are worthy and deserving of self care and that our needs are equally important.

One of my favorite quotes is from Maya Angelou: "If I am not good to myself, how can I expect anyone else to be good to me?" If we want to be treated differently, we must treat ourselves with grace and love first. And that's where self care comes into the conversation. Self care is vital for boosting self-confidence, maintaining good health, increasing your productivity and focus, and lowering your stress levels. When we take care of ourselves, we are at our best to take care of others, whether that is being a parent, interacting with co-workers, or running our own businesses.

Just when I needed it the most, another good friend introduced me to essential oils and the power of self care. I started using an immune-protective blend on the bottoms of my feet, and I added it to my diffuser. I used this blend faithfully every day, and after only a few weeks, I suddenly realized that I felt better. Not just better—*really* better. I was sleeping deeply. I had more energy. I wasn't moody. I felt like my old self again. I was *stunned*. Especially since it was wintertime, when germs abound, and it was the first time in twenty years that I didn't get sick. (And I didn't get sick for over three years!)

That was my first experience with essential oils, beyond getting an occasional massage, and I was like, "Holy moly, this stuff really works!" I even became a bit disappointed that no one had ever taken the time to really look for the root cause of my problem or suggest that I try essential oils. But I had to be sure that they were a legitimate answer to my prayers, while the science nerd in me needed to know the "why" behind this miracle cure. I used my biochemistry training to research the science and the chemical properties of the plants from which the oils were made. I studied dozens of books on essential oils and pored over hundreds of peer-reviewed articles.

Since this particular oil blend had helped to boost my immune system, what else were these oils capable of? Could they help with sleep? With tension in the head and neck? To detox us from some of the chemicals we use in our homes?

A resounding YES! This became the answer to all my questions and more. And this is because essential oils are adaptogenic. *Adaptogens* are plant substances that help us adapt to the internal and external environmental factors that cause stress. They support our body's systems, including hormonal balance, moods, the immune system, and overall homeostasis. They can be calming or energizing, grounding or uplifting, while affecting our body on a cellular level. They work quickly and effectively. Inhaling an essential oil allows it to penetrate the bloodstream through the respiratory system while triggering a response in the brain.

In addition to research on essential oils, I spent time learning the dirty secrets behind toxins lurking in our daily lives. Everything from the food we eat to the air we breathe, from the beauty products we apply to the medicines we take, could be harming our cellular and hormone function. I did a major life purge. I dumped anything I suspected was negatively affecting my hormones, especially the beauty products and cleansers that disrupted my hormone levels, cognitive function, and weight. I began to make my own natural solutions using essential oils and natural ingredients. My husband and I started using oils for almost everything in our household—either applying them topically or breathing them in. Oils became one of the first things I reached for in the morning and one of the last things I diffused before going to bed. Essential oils quickly became a foundational component of my productive and rewarding life.

For my patients, I started making my own synergistic essential oil blends. These patients showed immediate improvement. Inexpensive, easily portable, and intoxicatingly aromatic, essential oils enabled my patients to take charge of their own health care and begin to heal themselves. Whether for sleep or mood, libido or hormones, there seemed to be an essential oil for everything! While there wasn't an immediate solution to specifically boost estrogen or progesterone levels, I discovered that the oils helped create a balance in the body that would allow hormonal levels to reset. My patients were creating habits that they could rely on, that they could trust, and that gave them confidence in their bodies again.

Part of my teaching process was about the importance of rituals that reinforced all the new positive habits these women were bringing into their lives. These rituals help us to care for ourselves and spend time refocusing while enjoying the process. I taught them about mindfulness as well, because at the foundation of everything I've learned and incorporated into my protocol is that if we can't recognize our patterns and don't have self-empowering habits in place, we aren't going to feel better. Instead, we end up right back where we started—overwhelmed, stressed, and with our hormones out of whack.

I was not only empowering these women; I was also doing it myself. These lifestyle changes and rituals became an enormous part of my own learning process: I finally figured out that loving myself was the key to being able to give my best to my patients, my family, and my *everything*.

Essential oils enabled me to manage my stress load, be mindful of what I eat, carefully select appropriate supplements for my needs, and choose appropriate exercise for my body. Breathing techniques and daily rituals provided me with a solution for finding the calm amid a busy and stressful world. The oils support my lifestyle choices and sustain my well-being.

And now it's your turn to use this book as a tool to balance your life, with easy and practical solutions that you can implement for immediate results!

How to Use This Book

The best way to naturally create hormonal balance is by resetting your body's major systems through focused and deliberate changes in your daily habits, aided every step of the way by high-quality essential oils. Getting to the root cause of hormonal imbalance takes some time and introspection, but this book will give you a step-by-step system to balance your hormones and leave you feeling energized, joyful, and revitalized.

In Part I, "A Hormone and Essential Oil Primer," you will learn what hormones are, what their roles are in our body, and how they become unbalanced. Then we will explore the scientific basis of how essential oils work from a physiological aspect to reset and improve hormonal levels, and why they can mitigate the toxic load that we're carrying—and likely don't even know exists. The specific therapeutic properties of the oils most commonly used to solve hormonal symptoms will be introduced, and you will learn how to best use different essential oils for each; and in one of my favorite chapters, you'll find out how to create everyday rituals with essential oils to enhance your health and well-being.

Part II, "Using Essential Oils to Address Your Hormonal Symptoms," will present practical applications for immediate use in your life. The ten chapters are organized by topic, so you can quickly turn to them to address any of your issues. The solutions you'll find in these chapters are designed to work with your unique biochemistry, and are adaptive to your specific needs.

With over 100 recipes for essential oil blends created for this book, you will be able to easily locate and implement specific solutions for your individualized needs. Plus, they are so incredibly easy to concoct and use, your friends may start begging you for advice!

Part III, "The 14-Day Rescue Plan to Jump-Start Your Hormonal Health," is the ultimate guide to resetting your hormones and drastically improving your health. I'll get you ready with daily solutions and amazing rituals *before* you start, so you'll be able to focus during the step-by-step program with meal plans, exercise recommendations, rituals, and supportive essential oils for the following two weeks. You will be astonished by how much weight you may lose, how much better you will feel, and how easy it is to incorporate smart choices into your life for a powerful transformation with lasting results.

For example, when my energy is about to crash, I used to panic and think, *How do I fix this? What do I have? What can I eat?*

Now, my brain has reprogrammed me to say, *Okay, where are my oils?* I've learned to keep them by my side at all times. When I'm working on a big project at the computer for hours and my brain is about to shut down in a zombie-like state, I stand up, inhale an energy-booster blend made from a combination of Wild Orange and Peppermint for thirty seconds, apply a dab of Peppermint oil to my wrists, and do a short burst of exercise like jumping jacks or marching in place for a minute or two. Then, I add my Wake Up and Focus Diffuser Blend (page 146) to my diffuser, and I am totally myself again. Even *better*, I'd say. I am refreshed, energized, empowered, and ready to get back to work.

My mission is to impact the lives of all women who struggle with hormonal issues. I hope this book will do for you what essential oils have done for me. It's incredibly empowering when we take ownership of our own health.

Only *you* have the power to change your future, to take the reins of your own health and wellness and give your mind and body the attention and care that they deserve. Don't live another day suffering from your current "normal"—use this book to banish your hormone woes for good and transform your life.

PART I

A Hormone and Essential Oil Primer

CHAPTER 1

How to Balance Your Hormones Without Adding Hormones

H ow did I get here?

Many women find themselves in a hormonal crisis at some point in their lives, and they seek advice from medical professionals who, more likely than not, downplay common symptoms like depression, anxiety, weight gain, and brain fog in their failure to see the woman as a whole. Our unique history, genetic makeup, personality, emotional health, lifestyle, habits, and many more factors play into who we are, of course. We need to see beyond the surface—*who we are* is just as important as *what we present as*. We are not merely our symptoms. This is why I believe we must treat the *whole* person.

Society pressures women to be all things, all the time. It's not just about looking good, though we must do that, too. With a smile on our faces, looking our best, and with a pleasant and nurturing attitude, we navigate life not only for ourselves but also for our families, our friends, our co-workers, for those around us. We spend our lives taking care of our families and are often ostracized for it.

When we go back to work after having children, there is even less time to focus on and take care of ourselves. We neglect. We ignore. We push onward. And eventually our health takes a big toll.

Sadly, the timing often corresponds to when our hormonal levels begin to naturally decline and our bodies change as a result. An easy solution is to blame how badly we're feeling on our hormones. Sure, hormones are at play here, but you *can't* fix hormones with hormones. In fact, pumping in additional hormones may do more damage than good.

A holistic approach to identifying and understanding *who* you are as a woman, and then taking a hard look at the routines and lifestyle that landed you in your current predicament, must be done. Resetting your lifestyle with self-care routines and rituals supported by essential oils will help you to heal yourself. *You* know who *you* are better than anyone else, but learning how you got where you are, what you can do to reverse the problem, and identifying triggers that bring out symptoms will all be a part of your game plan.

So, if you are asked the question, "Are you hormonal?" you don't have to be offended. The answer is *yes*. We are *always* hormonal! Hormones keep our bodies functioning the way that they're designed to.

What we need to focus on is the ever-fluctuating balance of hormones in our own, unique system. No one solution will work for everyone, but a foundation of daily self-care rituals coupled with essential oils will help you discover the solutions you need. You just have to be willing to put in a little bit of work. Time to roll up your sleeves and get your body back.

Hormonal Basics

Hormones are not just about periods and hot flashes. Hormones are chemical messengers constantly at play in our bodies. They affect nearly all functions—influencing, triggering, and regulating everything from temperature to heartbeat, from blood sugar to fertility, from mood to sleep rhythms. The interconnectedness of all our body's systems makes it nearly impossible to isolate one hormone or one symptom and blame it for all our problems, since the body functions as a complex entity. What I have found in my years of practice is that women usually need to pay attention to several hormones. You need to assess your unique situation to create a personalized plan to reverse imbalances and reset your body.

What many of us don't realize, though, is that hormones work hard to keep our body in homeostasis, relaying important information as they convey messages from your brain to different organs. Basically, everything that we do causes hormonal fluctuations.

Where Do Hormones Come From?

The endocrine system, composed of a variety of specialized glands, is responsible for synthesizing and secreting hormones. Other organs contain endocrinocytes that also produce hormones, though that's not their main function. So while most people know that the reproductive system produces hormones, we sometimes ignore the important function of our adrenal glands, thyroid, and pancreas. In addition, organs involved in hormone production include the heart, kidneys, stomach and intestines, liver, and skin. Interestingly, even our adipose tissue, or fat, plays a role in the secretion and release of certain hormones.

In this book, I will primarily be focusing on hormones associated with metabolism, reproduction, the thyroid, and the HPA axis (hypothalamic-pituitary-adrenal axis), as they are the ones that tend to become imbalanced over time. Rebooting these hormones seems to clear out the body to heal itself with support from high-quality essential oils and key lifestyle changes.

The Reproductive System Hormones

Our reproductive years are the post-puberty years of menstruation and fertility, followed by the gradually decreasing hormonal levels of the perimenopausal phase, before arriving at menopause, clinically defined as the period following one full year of no menstruation. Your reproductive system is still functioning pre-puberty and post-menopause, but in a different way. Perhaps it was named the "reproductive" system since its primary and most incredible job is creating more humans. This is how a healthy reproductive system should function if all conditions are optimal:

ESTROGEN

Produced primarily by the ovaries, *estrogen* is the term used to refer to any compounds producing estrus: estrone, estradiol, and estriol. These three hormones directly affect a woman's growth and development, as well as regulate her reproductive system—namely, her menstrual cycle. Estrogen is also produced by the feto-placental unit during pregnancy, and in smaller amounts by the adrenal cortex and in the male testes.

PROGESTERONE

Progesterone production takes place in three main arenas: the ovaries during menstruation, the placenta during pregnancy, and the adrenal glands. Primarily responsible for preparing the uterus for conception and implantation, it aids in the regulation of the menstrual cycle and also helps to maintain viable pregnancies. When a new egg is produced each month and begins to develop in the follicle, estrogen and progesterone are both produced.

TESTOSTERONE

Though considered to be mainly a male hormone, testosterone is also produced in the female ovaries and adrenal glands. It influences bone strength and muscle mass and is essential to a woman's libido.

What Reproductive Hormones Do During Fertility

Estrogen and progesterone are the hormones responsible for creating optimal conditions for reproduction. *Estrogen* allows for a soft and thick uterine lining in days one to fourteen of a monthly cycle, before the egg is released for potential conception. It also tells our bodies to keep some extra fat around in case conception takes place so that we can protect the growing fetus. *Progesterone* is produced after ovulation by the corpus luteum (the sac that the egg comes from) and dominates the second half of the cycle (luteal phase). Its main job is to keep that comfy uterine lining in place for implantation of a fertilized egg. If this happens, levels continue to rise to ensure the uterine lining remains intact until the placenta is fully developed enough to take over, around twelve weeks into the pregnancy.

Each of us is born with a finite number of eggs. They are released monthly for potential fertilization and implantation. If conception does not take place, progesterone levels will decline, causing the uterine lining to shed—and our menstrual period to begin.

Sadly, many women experience debilitating premenstrual syndrome (PMS), or horrible periods, and symptoms that they attribute to normal hormone function. This is inaccurate. Your body is not supposed to suffer through its normal processes, but if hormone levels are out of whack (and not just the reproductive hormones), the results can trigger these painful conditions.

What Reproductive Hormones Do During Perimenopause

Usually around age forty, although sometimes as early as thirty-five, most women begin experiencing changes in their bodies associated with perimenopause, the period when childbearing comes to an end. Estrogen production specifically for the reproductive system gradually slows; eggs aren't always released every month and menstrual periods may become irregular. Our bodies slowly adapt over a period from four to ten years as we settle into the normal aging process. The last two years before menopause are when most women notice the biggest change, as hormone levels drop more steadily than before in preparation for cessation of the cycle entirely.

During this time, several changes happen owing to the decline in estrogen production. As estrogen influences bone density, attention to bone health becomes paramount. In addition, we use energy differently, and caloric needs shift so we can properly fuel our bodies and prevent weight gain and excess fat storage.

What Reproductive Hormones Do During Menopause

After your period has ceased for one year, you are officially in menopause, the culmination of perimenopausal changes. Ovarian production of hormones ceases entirely, but the adrenal glands continue to produce them for the body's needs. Any perimenopausal symptoms usually decline and disappear at this stage. Women become more at risk for chronic conditions such as heart disease and osteoporosis/osteopenia during post-menopause.

Thyroid Hormones

Known as the "butterfly gland" because of its unique shape, the thyroid sits at the front of the neck, where it regulates hundreds of functions, particularly our metabolic function, growth, and easing the body into maturity. The thyroid depends on iodine, a trace element not produced naturally in the body, and good diet to properly function. Iodine from food consumption is converted to produce the protein thyroglobulin, which is then converted into T4 (thyroxine) and other hormones.

TSH (Thyroid-Stimulating Hormone). Produced by the pituitary gland, TSH stimulates the production of T4 (thyroxine) and T3 (triiodothyronine).

T3 (Triiodothyronine). Converted from T4 via the liver and other tissues, T3 is the active form of thyroid hormone that affects metabolic processes, weight, energy, memory, cholesterol, muscle strength, heart rate, menstrual cycle, and more.

T4 (Thyroxine). Secreted by the thyroid gland directly into the bloodstream, T4 is an inactive thyroid hormone that functions as a storage component for T3. Levels of T4 in the body trigger the production or cessation of TSH.

Reverse T3 (RT3). An inactive form of T3 is produced when the body saves energy in the T4–T3 conversion process. Low levels can lead to hypothyroidism, while too much results in the blockage of T3 from its receptors.

What Thyroid Hormones Do

Optimal levels of T3 and T4 increase our basal metabolic rate (BMR), causing our bodies to kick into action. Body temperature rises while the heart rate quickens, and our body uses up energy a lot faster. The thyroid taps into the liver and muscles for stored energy in order to support functions like growth and development.

Often described as a "thermostat system," the hypothalamus functions as the adjuster of the thermostat, the pituitary gland. When the temperature—T3 and T4 levels—drops too low in the body, the hypothalamus releases TSH-Releasing Hormone (TRH), which tells the pituitary gland that it had better heat things up. As a result, the pituitary produces TSH, which triggers production of

T4 and ups the temperature. Sensing the shift, the pituitary lowers production of TSH and the system maintains balance.

The HPA Axis Hormones

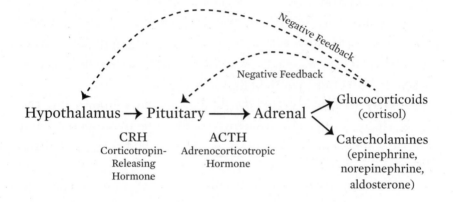

HYPOTHALAMUS

The hypothalamus regulates the autonomic nervous system, sending messages directly from the brain to various areas of the body, including the thyroid, pituitary, and adrenal glands, as well as other organs. It maintains our sleep cycles and appropriate energy levels, regulates body temperature, and influences our appetite, thirst, weight, moods (such as anger and fear), blood pressure, and libido.

PITUITARY GLAND

The pituitary gland sits at the base of the brain, physically connected to the hypothalamus. Considered the master control gland in the body, it produces a wide variety of hormones, directly triggers the thyroid and adrenal cortex, and influences the reproductive system and kidney function.

ADRENAL GLANDS

The pair of adrenal glands sit atop the kidneys, where they produce hormones to help regulate blood sugar, energy storage, the immune system, and metabolism. From steroids to stress to sex, the adrenals keep our bodies safe and primed for whatever scenario might ensue.

What HPA Axis Hormones Do

The complexity of the body's systems never ceases to amaze me, and the HPA axis really gets the science nerd in me excited! The interconnectedness and interplay among such tiny molecules of our body demonstrates the sheer power of big things in small packages. But it doesn't take much to push these delicate balances into overload or completely throw them off-balance.

Responsible for a variety of bodily processes, the HPA axis directly influences digestion, the immune system, energy storage and expenditure, and mood and emotional responses. The claim to fame for the adrenals, however, is their ability to respond to stress.

The primary function of the HPA axis is to keep the body on an even keel, so it activates when exposed to a potential stressor—a short-term stress response. It all begins in the hypothalamus, which perceives the stressor and begins to produce CRH (corticotropin-releasing hormone) to tell the pituitary gland that something is posing a potential threat. The pituitary responds with production of ACTH (adrenocorticotropic hormone), kicking the adrenal glands into action. They then respond to the stressor by having the body produce several different hormones for our own protection.

The catecholamine *epinephrine* (aka adrenaline) raises heart rate and increases blood pressure, getting us ready for a potential fight-or-flight scenario: we either fight off the tiger or run for our lives. It also dilates our respiratory passages, allowing for greater airflow to oxygenate our bodies for the battle. The adrenals also produce the glucocorticoid *cortisol*, which raises our blood sugar levels in order to fuel this ensuing battle, with the help of adrenaline that aids the liver in the conversion of glycogen (think stored energy) into glucose (fuel for the body). It also redirects the body's attention away from unnecessary systems at the time in favor of survival, so digestion and reproduction take a back seat in favor of saving our own lives.

When we perceive the stressor to be eliminated, the body triggers a negative feedback from the adrenals to the pituitary and hypothalamus so that they slow their production of ACTH and CRH. This returns the body to a normal balance and life goes on.

How Hormonal Imbalance Happens and Its Resulting Symptoms

Though our bodies are constantly bombarded from every angle externally, the way it responds *internally* often creates our hormonal imbalances. In my years of practice, I have found stress to be the single biggest cause for hormonal imbalance among women, owing to the interconnectedness of all our systems. What was meant to be a complex mechanism for keeping our bodies in top condition can easily tip into an out-of-whack, imbalanced mess, triggering multiple symptoms and leaving us asking that fateful question: *How did I get here?*

That is the exact question thirty-eight-year-old Rita, a single mother, asked me within minutes of walking into my office. Suffering from chronic fatigue, she looked panicked and exhausted, and struggled to get out of bed each morning. She barely had enough energy in the morning to make her daughter's lunch and get to her demanding job on time—a job that left her feeling overworked and underappreciated. She had substituted self care and healthy food choices with long nights at the office and trips to Starbucks. Once we figured out the core issue, we worked together to get her body and energy back on track.

If we look at the short-term stress functioning of the HPA axis and apply chronic, unrelenting stress to it, our bodies take on an entirely new landscape. Instead of managing the stress and slowing the hormonal response through the negative feedback loop, our hypothalamus becomes overwhelmed with perceived stress. In our modern world, stress could be anything from driving in heavy traffic each day, to taxing job responsibilities, to advertisements reminding us we haven't planned for retirement yet. Or, it can be a comment a co-worker says to us, sending us into a whirlwind of worry or frustration.

Chronic Stress = Adrenal Stress

Unrelenting stress from every angle continuously triggers the HPA axis until it is overworked and under cared for. Swamped with excess levels of cortisol, the body senses it's in a "My Body at War" state, with danger lurking around every corner. As a result, temporary shutdowns of unnecessary systems become more permanent situations, causing an onslaught of symptoms:

- Decreased metabolic function triggers starvation mode to save energy for the upcoming battles. We need fewer calories when this happens, but we often continue to eat whatever is available, making it much harder to lose weight.
- There is weight gain in the "inner tube" pattern around the middle, as well as around vital organs and in adipose tissue to store energy. This increases belly fat.
- Muscle mass declines as the body attacks them to get glucose for energy to battle the threat.
- Binge eating becomes commonplace because we are feeding an unmet need, in the form of stress or emotional distress. Add that to our habit of scarfing food as quickly as possible to move to the next task, and eating becomes a survival mechanism.
- Pseudo-famine situations trigger midnight binges and comfort-food cravings, because carbs and sugar are what we really need as fuel when our lives are being threatened.
- Increased sugar consumption overloads the body and creates unnatural highs and crashes, much like a drug addiction.

- Reproduction is put on hold in favor of survival, because the body wouldn't allow a baby to come into the world where there is no food and perpetual danger lurking around every corner. Bring on infertility, irregular periods, PMS symptoms, and more.
- Exhaustion and brain fog from chronic stress and lack of sleep become the new normal.

And the stressors keep on coming. These symptoms are just the beginning of hormonal imbalance, and can eventually lead to scarier conditions, like Type 2 diabetes, autoimmune conditions, and heart disease.

Now, let's address what I'll discuss in the Five Pillars of a Foundational Lifestyle section in Part III.

First off are nutritional deficiencies. If you haven't been fueling your body properly, it can't possibly get the nutrients it needs to function optimally. Add in lack of exercise to keep your muscles primed, your heart rate normalized, and your body in top condition (especially to combat the excess amounts of stress), and you have a real problem.

And that's not all, because there are factors out of your control that affect your body, such as environmental toxins lurking in the air, water, the food you eat, the containers you store food in and cook it in, the products that you apply to your skin, and the medicines that you are prescribed or buy at the drugstore.

Where does that leave you? In a danger state, for sure—but don't lose hope! There is a way to reverse the damage, rebalance your body, and recharge your life to increase your vitality and renew your sense of self.

Do I Need a Reboot?

Chances are, if you picked up this book and are still reading, you need a reboot. Or you know something is off and you're desperate to figure out a solution.

I know. I was there, too.

Here's the good news: you CAN do this! Are there specific signs and signals letting you know that your body is hormonally imbalanced? Yes!

I created a quiz that I give to all my patients to see just how *off* their bodies may be owing to hormonal or other issues. They are almost always surprised by the results. I can't tell you how many times patients have told me they are healthy, yet they check off nearly all (if not all!) the boxes.

Given how polluted our environment is, how overloaded with chemicals our food is, and how unhealthy our diets can be, it's almost impossible to live without any health issues at all. There are just too many external factors working against us. Instead, what you want to strive for is the best possible health you can have, given all the mitigating factors you face. Being mindful of how well you take care of yourself on a day-to-day basis is a start. And supporting your changes with the power and potency of essential oils will keep you empowered to succeed.

The Comprehensive Hormone Quiz

The Comprehensive Hormone Quiz was designed to provide you with a snapshot of your hormonal imbalances so you can begin implementing essential oils, self-care rituals, and better lifestyle habits to get your body back on track. Before heading into Part II, go to www.drmariza .com/hormonequiz to take the quiz and figure out the root cause of your hormonal imbalance.

The Role of Your Trusted Health-Care Provider

It's very important that your personal health-care provider understands and supports your hormonal issues without denigrating or dismissing them. If you aren't getting the support you need, ask friends or colleagues for recommendations. Remember, *you* need to advocate for your own wellness. You have the right to demand proper testing and evaluation. It can be daunting for many of us to advocate for ourselves, as we aren't used to taking health-care matters into our own hands—but it's time to begin!

So, while some doctors combine traditional medicine with a holistic approach seamlessly, you may need to turn elsewhere for support in areas like nutrition, essential oils, supplementation, and natural hormone balance. Be proactive in seeking out a support team with whom you feel comfortable. A team can be very effective as long as there is clear communication about your protocols and recommendations. Look for functional practitioners, naturopaths, chiropractors, and other holistic health-care providers. Most of them should be able to order and competently address any testing results and recommendations. I have provided some trusted sources to help you find an integrative or functional practitioner in the Resources section of this book.

I recommend these tests for everyone dealing with a potential hormone imbalance. Do your research and read about each one if it makes you feel more comfortable. You need to be on board with this plan before we can begin our journey to success and balance.

The Testing You Need

The secret sauce to testing is to measure hormonal levels and expect improvements over time. Ask your integrative or functional doctor to order the following:

- A complete blood panel
- Thyroid tests: TSH, Free T3, Free T4, Reverse T3 (RT3), TPOAb, AntiTgAntibody
- Adrenal tests: Measure serum cortisol first thing in the morning, before 9 a.m., four diurnal cortisol (tested four times during the day via saliva), free and total testosterone, and dehydroepiandrosterone (DHEA)
- Progesterone on day 21–23 (if you're cycling)
- Fasting insulin and glucose, HDL, and hemoglobin A1C
- IGF-1 (growth hormone)
- 25-hydroxy-vitamin D, vitamin B_{12}, folate

For a complete list of lab tests, test descriptions and optimal ranges for each test, head over to www.drmariza.com/labtests.

If your doctor won't order these blood tests, order them yourself. Find a source for trusted laboratories in the Resources (page 351).

When you assess the test results, pay attention to the "normal ranges." Discuss them with your trusted healthcare provider, and bear in mind that just because your number falls into the "normal" range, that doesn't mean that it's normal for *you*. Any number at the higher or lower end should be questioned.

What Essential Oils Can and Can't Do

In my time as a health-care practitioner, I have researched, studied, and recommended a variety of protocols to my patients, none of which revolutionized their success like essential oils. The immediate support that they offer is unparalleled, which is why they've been used for hundreds of years for their potency and power. I'll never forget my first whiff of Wild Orange essential oil and the immediate uplift I felt.

But before we get into what essential oils *can* do, let me take a minute to explain what they *can't* do.

Even though essential oils exhibit specialized properties and are composed of hundreds of potent constituents, they are *not* hormones! Essential oils can't become hormones. They can't produce hormones. They can't replace hormones. Nature just doesn't work that way.

But—nature gave us these amazing gifts that *can* support our bodies in healing themselves and that affect our bodies in miraculous ways. In other words, you can *treat* hormones without hormones. Essential oils are your support. Use them as tools to get you to the endgame: healthy hormonal levels. But they won't get you there alone if you neglect lifestyle choices that establish the foundation for your good health.

How Essential Oils Support Hormones Without Adding Hormones

The amazing power of essential oils can support your body to get its hormone-balancing systems back into a stable balance. Scientific studies continue to support essential-oil science in making new breakthroughs and in discovering the power of how their constituents influence the body. Sometimes I think we are a bit late in the game, since these gifts of nature have been used for thousands of years, especially in Eastern medicine—but better late than never!

Bridging the Gap—The Five Pillars of a Foundational Lifestyle

I am always astounded by our body's ability to function and heal, even under stressful circumstances. Think about the last time you worried about a cut on your finger closing up and healing— probably never. Your cells collaborate to heal your cut without your even asking.

As you can imagine, the interconnectedness of the human body elements is remarkably complex. Add that to the intricacies of our hormonal makeup, and you've got a real miracle!

But your cells need your help. The very best and the most consistent daily habits can make all the difference in how you feel—and especially how your body functions. It's the difference between your feeling wired and tired throughout the day or experiencing boundless energy.

As you know, I learned the hard way that poor daily habits can create significant cellular imbalance if you let yourself slip too far. I have a feeling that's why you are reading this book right now!

The Five Pillars outlined here and described in more detail in Chapter 15 support our very being, hold us up when times get rough, and keep us balanced and strong. But if we neglect them over time, they will begin to erode, crumble, and even work against us, causing internal problems that often don't break the surface until it's too late for a simple solution. The longer you ignore the destruction, pushing past the symptoms or naively accepting them as your "normal," the more difficult your reboot and recovery will be.

When our bodies are imbalanced and underserved, it is almost as if they begin to resist the changes we try to institute. This is why there is no overnight solution to this problem. While you can get instantaneous relief from using essential oils, using them in isolation while you continue to allow the icebergs to exist is pointless. They will not help you to bridge the gaps; they will simply provide a light bandage for your problems, fulfilling an immediate need to ease the symptoms much the way many over-the-counter drugs simply mask symptoms.

The combination of essential-oil support and lifestyle changes is what will get you back on track—*but only if you are willing to make the changes and allow them time to work.* Acknowledging that these Five Pillars need some rebuilding is the first step in your rebooting process to the best possible you. After all, your body can only do so much with so little.

Pillar #1—Nutrition

THE PROBLEM

By failing to properly fuel our bodies and falling into patterns of poor, imbalanced nutrition, we unknowingly create a downward spiral of hormonal imbalance from which it is hard to recover.

Addressing nutritional imbalances and deficiencies with a whole-food diet and supplementation will ensure that your body gets back into balance. Nothing is going to help you unless you realize that *what* you eat matters just as much as *how much* you eat. Think of food as information for your body—you want to convey the right information to your cells and organs.

THE ESSENTIAL-OILS SOLUTION

Essential oils can help you to resist the cravings that have you conditioned to eat unhealthy choices, can support your body in losing excess weight, and can enhance your overall vitality. Thus, Chapter 8 focuses on weight gain caused by hormonal imbalance; Chapter 13 discusses digestive issues that may be plaguing you on a daily basis. And the 14-Day Rescue Plan, in Part III, is the final fix that will enable you to rework your nutritional choices so that food works *for* you, fueling your needs in the way your body appreciates.

Pillar #2—Exercise

THE PROBLEM

When your hormones are out of whack, your normal exercise routine may not help you recover, and in some cases, may even make you feel worse.

THE ESSENTIAL-OILS SOLUTION

Essential oils not only help your body to recover from the symptoms of hormonal issues but can also enable your body to re-center itself over time. In addition, they can greatly support your body during pre- and post-exercise routines, as well as speed up your recovery time after exercise.

Chapter 5 covers the far-reaching damage that sustained cortisol levels from stress can do on your body; energy and fatigue are addressed in Chapter 6; Chapter 8 dives into weight gain and the cravings that often fuel it. The role of female hormones is covered in Chapter 9. And you'll see how to do the best exercises to tackle hormonal chaos in the 14-Day Rescue Plan, which is in Part III.

Pillar #3—Stress Management

THE PROBLEM

Chronic, elevated levels of cortisol and other hormones can chip away at your body's systems, causing them to weaken one by one until you can have major health issues.

THE ESSENTIAL-OILS SOLUTION

Studies have shown that, when cortisol levels are high, inhaling essential oils can calm the mind and relax the body.

In Chapter 5, you'll read about the damage stress can do; Chapter 11 focuses on the fluctuation of emotions in a woman's life and how they can lead you into a downward spiral of hormonal disaster; and Chapter 12 examines cognition, and how brain fog and an inability to concentrate affect your life.

Pillar #4—Reducing the Toxic Burden

THE PROBLEM

Many people are shocked when they learn about how a toxic load can affect their cellular function, especially when it's the result of decades of chemicals and toxins stressing the body.

Strong scientific evidence links dangerous toxins and synthetics in personal-care products to chronic diseases, reproductive toxicity, autoimmunity, allergies, and cancer.

THE ESSENTIAL-OILS SOLUTION

Nutritional changes will help rid your body of toxins from food, but ridding your environment of as many other toxins as possible, including those you put on your body, must become a top priority. Learning to make your own products that are free of harmful toxins, diffusing essential oils to cleanse the air, and unleashing the power of essential oils are all paramount in reversing as many of these effects as possible. Chapter 8 explains how even your weight can be influenced by toxins in the food you eat; Chapter 14 discusses the effects of toxicity and focuses on showing how you can make your own all-natural beauty and cleaning products.

Pillar #5—Self-Care Rituals

THE PROBLEM

In a world where women are expected to do it all, often at the expense of their own health, they are quick to put themselves last. If you aren't the best possible version of yourself, then you are potentially neglecting everything you are trying to balance.

THE ESSENTIAL-OILS SOLUTION

Imagine the impact you could have on all your desires if you truly felt good from the inside out. Spending time caring for yourself allows you to support everyone and everything else in your life. Essential oils can help you find that balance.

In Chapter 7, you will learn how to improve your sleep; Chapter 10 focuses on libido and recharging the energy in the bedroom. Chapter 11 addresses emotional health, keeping you empowered and positive, especially if your symptoms were misdiagnosed as mental health issues when they actually were caused by hormonal imbalances. And Chapter 15 will give you even more details about self-care rituals.

Essential Oils Transformed My Life

Throughout this book, I share my own struggles with hormonal imbalance and describe the crumbling foundation that was my life. I want you to know that you're not alone, that you are not the only one silently suffering. But you can no longer gloss over the increasing symptoms and ignore the new ones as they surface. The help you seek is in these pages. I honestly cannot imagine my life without my daily use of essential oils. I quickly fell in love with their amazing power, and their immediate effect on my body at a cellular level. For you as well, they can provide the same relief as I desired for so long, while supporting your body's ability to heal itself.

Unlike many over-the-counter and prescribed remedies, essential oils not only affect the body systemically but also can be used quite frequently. This means not needing to wait thirty minutes for a medication to circulate through your system. It also means not masking a symptom. Rather, it means supporting your body in healing from the inside out. It also means, however, that for them to work, you need a major reboot, identifying those foundational issues and symptoms that have plagued you the most. You start by putting yourself first and shifting your belief to self care.

Empowering women to love and honor their bodies has become my mission. Supported by the amazing power of essential oils, I have helped thousands of women find personal successes. No matter what point you're at in your life, you need support to heal yourself and time devoted to self care. Only then will you be truly able to give your all to others and to what you enjoy doing. Let's rebuild our foundation, kick the symptoms to the curb, bridge the gaps, and discover how amazing we feel when we rebalance, recharge, and revitalize our lives!

CHAPTER 2

The Guide to Using Essential Oils

Starting out in the world of essential oils can be overwhelming, and there is definitely a learning curve involved—which will be a lot easier when you know the specifics before you oil up for the first time.

When I first came in contact with essential oils, I adored the uplifting and perky scent of Wild Orange essential oil. Phototoxicity, dilution, and ingestion were topics that never crossed my mind; it was truly love at first scent. Now I know to always do my homework before using any essential oil.

Guided selection, proper usage technique, and safety precautions must be considered prior to launching your essential-oil journey. Let me be your guide as we take a walk through the basics.

How to Choose an Essential Oil

Essential oils seem to be popping up everywhere, with varying brands, different claims, and every bottle labeled that its oil is "pure." I can assure you that it just isn't the case. For starters, there aren't strict regulations governing the packaging of essential oils in this country, leading to a lot of companies selling highly adulterated oils that will not yield your desired results and could potentially harm your body with whatever solvents or chemicals lurk inside the bottle. They may be cheaper, but the cheap oils do not meet the quality standards I require of my essential oils.

Please also know that the blends, protocols, and advice I give in this book concern *only* high-quality essential oils from respected, trusted companies that adhere to certain quality standards. (Using my suggestions with lesser-quality oils just won't be as effective, so you'll be wasting your time and money. But don't just take my word for it. Do your own research to learn the basics and to find a company that practices the safety and quality standards you can trust.)

Why are these lesser-quality oils significantly less effective? Because they aren't meant for therapeutic benefits and they don't meet high-quality, scientific testing standards. There are different grades of oils, and 98 percent of the essential oils currently produced fall into one of two categories: food grade or perfume grade. In addition to being heavily adulterated with additives and solvents, their main purpose is to provide a standard scent for their particular purpose. So, lavender soap always smells the same from Company A, while lemon cleaner always smells the same from Company B. Consumers know what to expect when they repurchase their favorite products—and that's a consistency in fragrance. Also, all-natural essential oils cannot be patented, but mainstream companies would rather use a synthetic version for medicines, perfumes, personal-care products, and foods.

In the United States, most perfume-grade oils sold as "pure" are simply fragrance-grade and diluted. But not just diluted with alcohol, water, or other oils. They also have been created with the use of synthetic chemicals—colorless, odorless solvents that will remain in your bottle of oil. You may find that your body immediately responds to these adulterated oils, or you develop symptoms over time. If you're only looking for the perfume results of these oils as fragrances for laundry, air fresheners, or cleaners, then adulteration may not be a problem. But I prefer not to have any sort of chemicals freely roaming in my environment and I would NEVER put them on my skin.

So, how do you know what you have? Start with the *Paper Test*: Put one drop of the questionable oil on a piece of paper. Let it sit and evaporate for an hour. If there is any ring or residue left behind, you have an adulterated oil. This test works for most essential oils such as Peppermint, Lemon, and Lavender. Note that this test won't work for Myrrh, Patchouli, and the rare absolutes like Jasmine, Rose, and Vanilla, which must be processed with solvents owing to their more delicate nature.

The companies I respect most and whose products I feel comfortable using pay close attention to where the oil-producing plants are grown, their harvest time, and the proper distillation, with care to temperature and length of time. It does concern me that there aren't more regulations, which is why the companies I trust set their own quality standards. For the highest-quality essential oils, the answer should be yes to the majority of the following questions you should ask of the producers:

- Does the company disclose where the oil is sourced?
- Do they take care to harvest at peak times to ensure the highest quality product?
- Do they use testing procedures to ensure potency and purity?
- Have they created partnerships with local growers and harvesters for a mutually beneficial relationship?
- Do they use sound business practices and are their leaders trustworthy?
- Are both gas chromatography and mass spectrometry tests done to ensure quality? (Both of these tests must be used to verify the presence of the correct compounds and to ensure that no impurities are present in the final product.)
- Is testing done for microbial properties?

There are steps you can take to ensure that what you already have on hand are high-quality essential oils, as well as to assess the oils you are considering purchasing.

Ten Assurances for High-Quality Essential Oils

1. **Names.** The common and scientific (Latin) names of the source plant should be clearly displayed on the label. If the oil is diluted, that should be labeled and the carrier oil should be listed. If it is a blend, every essential oil contained therein used should be listed, with its common and scientific names, as well as any carrier oils.

2. **ATI.** Each bottle should be labeled with the recommended usage guidelines for that particular oil: aromatic (A), topical (T), or internal (I). Sometimes directions may be written on the bottle, but most times the directions are simply labeled with these letters.

3. **Therapeutic Grade.** The grade should be clearly listed and/or advertised. This references the presence of each oil's primary constituents in proper form, as well as its health benefits. Companies producing high-quality essential oils usually have their own internal quality standards that indicate their process for ensuring their essential oils are pure, potent, and effective.

4. **Bottled and Capped.** The bottle should be dark glass (amber or cobalt) to protect from sun exposure, tightly capped, stored or presented upright, and fitted with an orifice reducer (a plastic insert that seals the top of the bottle and protects it from oxidation from air exposure). Dropper tops should only be added after you purchase the oil.

5. **Size.** Sizes for high-quality essential oils are usually 5-, 10-, or 15 mL, dispensed for use with an orifice reducer that produces drops. A 15-mL bottle of essential oil contains about 250 drops. It may not seem like a lot, but because you will only use one to two drops per recipe, the bottle usually lasts

quite a while, making it more cost-effective than its medicinal counterparts. When you consider cost per drop, essential oils are not expensive.

6. **Price.** Oils that are all priced the same are a giant red flag. Each oil requires a unique process of growing, harvesting, and extracting, as well as a different amount of plant material, so prices should always vary. For example, it takes approximately 105 pounds of rose petals to produce a 5-mL bottle of Rose essential oil—and we all know roses aren't cheap!

7. **Expiration Date.** Most high-quality essential oils offer an expiration date for shelf life, but this is because most have also been approved as food-grade and are stamped with the acronym GRAS (generally recognized as safe) in the United States for use in cooking. This doesn't mean that they are safe for internal usage as a supplement, however. At minimum, the expiration date gives you an indication of how long a bottle has been sitting on a shelf.

8. **Company.** Do you recognize the company name? Have you researched it and feel comfortable with what you found? Does it pass the suggested questions on page 39?

9. **Senses.** Smell the oil for a crisp, clean, and balanced scent. Feel the oil to see if it leaves a residue. Watch it on your skin for quick absorption into your skin with only a clean scent remaining. If the scent adversely affects you or the oils don't absorb, then proceed with caution.

10. **Potency.** How much do you have to use to achieve your desired results? If it's more than one or two diluted drops, you have a lesser-quality oil. If you use a lot and experience no results or have adverse effects such as skin irritations or other symptoms, you probably have a lesser-quality oil.

For websites that recommend where to buy high-quality, therapeutic-grade essential oils, see Resources.

How to Use Essential Oils

As mentioned, essential oils can be used in three different ways: aromatically, topically, or internally. Not all these methods are recommended for each oil, so be sure that you check the bottle for the recommended usage or follow my guidelines to ensure you are using them properly. All the recipes in this book should be used in one of these three ways. Remember that each person is different, and the essential oils may cause different responses. It probably will take some trials to find your preferred methods for using each oil or blend, but don't let this discourage you!

There are three main groups by which we classify essential oils based on their effects: calming/soothing, uplifting/energizing, and grounding/balancing. These should be guidelines for the effects you can expect when using a particular essential oil, and you will see me use these terms to describe the effects of oils I recommend in this book.

As always, discuss your implementation of essential oils in your routine with a trusted integrative health-care provider, or essential oil expert, especially if you have any preexisting conditions. That said, trust your gut and stand up for yourself if your practitioners roll their eyes at you. You may want to seek out a more holistic health-care practitioner who is accepting of alternative and Eastern forms of care, if your current provider isn't willing to work with your requests. You are the CEO of your own health care!

Using Essential Oil Blends

While harnessing the potency and power of a single essential oil is extremely beneficial, even more profound effects can be achieved by using more than one. After spending years researching the most effective combinations, I've created and tested protocols that have worked for my patients with great success, and they will definitely support you as well. You will see many recipes for essential oil blends in this book; each oil was selected for a specific reason, including consideration of its constituents and blending properties with the other suggested essential oils.

Whether you choose to inhale, diffuse, apply, layer, or ingest these essential oils, remember that you want to give them an honest try. Don't give up after one application or trial, as your body needs different things at different times, or it may need the oils to be applied in a certain location or layered in a particular order. Work with them and give each a chance to help you when you need it most.

Aromatic Uses

The easiest way to use essential oils is aromatically. Owing to their volatile nature, essential oils quickly evaporate and pervade an area, directly entering the lungs and the brain's olfactory system, where they stimulate olfactory receptors. Mitral cells then carry the output signals from the olfactory bulb to the limbic brain, which influences emotions, memory, sleep, and hormonal balance, as well as to other areas of the brain.

Even more amazingly, from a simple whiff, the oils absorb into your bloodstream, where they travel throughout your body, affecting the areas that need them most. The longer you expose the oils directly to air, the more intense effect and aroma you will experience. Eventually, they are excreted through the kidneys, lungs, and pores, after their amazing influence on your entire body. Most important, they can directly affect the endocrine system, responsible for much of our hormone production and the HPA axis to help you find and keep the balance that you need.

Under the "aromatic umbrella," there are several ways to use the essential oils: direct inhalation, indirect inhalation, steamers, and diffusion. Used topically, however, you will also experience aromatic benefits. I recommend giving each a try to see which method you prefer; you may find that you like certain blends to be diffused while for others you may want to crack the top of the bottle and take in a deep whiff. It's all about what works for you!

DIRECT INHALATION

Opening a bottle and inhaling easily introduces these powerful aromas into your body, affecting your emotions, mood, and other systems. Be careful not to put the bottle too close to your nose or eyes, though, as the vapors can be intense. As a general rule of thumb, hold the bottle an arm's length away and slowly bring it in, breathing deeply and pausing to assess the effects. Until you know how an oil affects you, take care not to overload your sense too quickly. Direct inhalation should always be the first way to use a new oil.

If all goes well with your initial test, you can move on to patch-testing the oil (see page 55). If you have no reactions, then you can use the palm inhalation method for direct inhalation. To do this, put a drop or two in your palms, rub them gently together, and then cup them over your nose and mouth before deeply breathing.

INDIRECT INHALATION

For this method, add one or two drops of essential oil to an object that will then allow a slower, sustained release of its aroma. A cotton ball or tissue strategically placed allows you to do so in specific locations. For example, try attaching a cotton ball or wooden clothespin to a fan or air vent, put a few drops directly on the filters of your air conditioner, or hide felt squares with oils in your car, drawers, gym bag, or purse. One of my favorite tricks is to put a drop or two on the scarf I'm wearing that day for a sustained effect. Everyone always comments on how good I smell and I reap the benefits of the aromatherapy—and so do those around me.

There are also many options for diffuser jewelry, from lava beads to diffuser lockets, chic leather bracelets to clay pendants. Why not accessorize with a boost of essential oils that are more potent and beneficial than any perfume you've ever tried? They also make amazing gifts, especially for those people in your life who may need an essential oil boost as well.

DIFFUSION

Diffusion or nebulizing diffusion generally refers to small devices that take the power of essential oils and create a fine airborne mist that fills a larger area. Though many people prefer sustained diffusion, I recommend only diffusing an hour at a time and then taking a break to give your systems a reset. Be sure to use care if you have a preexisting respiratory condition and discuss the use of a diffuser with your trusted health-care professional. Many people with respiratory difficulties have found great success with diffusers, but you always want to err on the side of caution, especially if you are using other medications to control your condition.

My favorite is an ultrasonic cool-air diffuser that uses ultrasonic vibrations to turn a water vapor/essential oil mixture into a fine airborne mist. The oils can then remain suspending in the air for several hours for sustained breathable benefits. You only need to add four to six drops of high-quality essential oil to about a cup of water and push the button.

Be sure to follow the manufacturer's suggestions on your diffuser for use and care. The diffuser recipes in this book were all created for an ultrasonic cool-air diffuser.

Other diffusers blow air through an oil-soaked pad, but this just doesn't do the job like an ultrasonic cool-air diffuser. Also, definitely avoid using a diffuser that has a heating element that comes into contact with any oil, which can break down the chemical constituents, thereby reducing the effectiveness of the oils. Avoid using humidifiers or vaporizers, since their components are not manufactured for use with essential oils; essential oils can break down the plastics and cause toxins to leach out into the air, eventually ruining the machine's parts.

Using Steam in Your Home

Steam can be a natural diffuser for essential oils when used in the right way. Adding a few drops of essential oil to a steamy mug of water and then inhaling deeply can also give you the therapeutic benefits of a diffuser without a machine. Or try a steamy shower. A spritz will open your airways, awaken your senses, and bring you to balance—you just need to add water and essential oils to a two-ounce spray bottle and keep it in the shower. For a recipe, see Chapter 6.

Topical Uses

Topical application of essential oils to the skin allows the chemical constituents to combine with the natural sebum of your skin for absorption into the body. From the lymphatic system to soft tissue, the oils penetrate deep into the body. Muscles, surrounding tissue, and all other surrounding areas receive the benefits as the essential oils make their way into the bloodstream and travel through the organs before being excreted. Also, by applying the oils to your skin, you get the aromatherapeutic bonus effect of breathing in their scent, too.

NEAT VS. DILUTED

Remember that the potency of pure, high-quality therapeutic essential oils requires only a drop (or less) to be used for maximum benefit. As a result, we generally talk with two terms when referring to topical application: neat and diluted.

Neat means applying the drop of oil directly to the skin from the bottle. While there are several essential oils I feel comfortable using neat, such as Lavender and Frankincense, I always recommend diluting essential oils to know how your body will react to them. If you happen to apply an oil neat, you can always dilute it quickly afterward or if a reaction develops with one of the preferred carrier oils mentioned on pages 50–51.

Dilution happens when you mix the essential oil with a high-quality carrier oil to keep it from evaporating too fast and to cover a larger area of the skin. The carrier oil also helps to prevent the potential of an adverse dermal reaction. While oils repel water, they are lipophilic with other natural oils and fatty substances, combining and blending well for topical application.

My favorite carrier oils include raw organic cold-pressed unrefined coconut oil (solid form), fractionated coconut oil (liquid form), jojoba, grapeseed, or sweet almond oil. Jojoba works the best for any application on your face, since it is the closest to your natural sebum. I use coconut oil and sweet almond oil more than any of the others owing to their light scent and additional benefits to the body. See more on carrier oils on pages 50–51.

WHERE TO APPLY ESSENTIAL OILS

The recipes this book provides recommend application locations and directions on how to apply. Though these are suggested locations that you should try first, you should also trust your gut and experiment to find the place or places that work best for you. Knowing your body is key to making essential oils work for you. In general, however, I always tell my patients the following:

Where Needed. The general rule for essential oils is to apply them directly or close to where the oil is needed. For example, if you are dealing with tension in your back, you could massage diluted Peppermint oil directly to the sore spot. However, if you are looking to alleviate a tension headache behind your eyes, you would never apply the oils directly to your eyes. Instead, opt for locations close to the eyes, such as on your forehead or your temples, since the oils will go where they are needed once absorbed.

Pulse Points. Behind the ears, on the neck, temples, wrists, ankles, and over your heart—these are all known as pulse points, or places where you can feel your heartbeat the strongest. They allow the essential oils to be quickly absorbed into the bloodstream, but are also ideal locations for aromatherapeutic benefits. You don't have to apply essential oils to all of them at the same time, though some women find that this works the best for them. Experiment with oils individually and in combinations to see what garners maximum results. For me, a magic spot is right behind my ears—I get the benefit of aromatherapy all day long while my body reaps the benefits. Other friends swear by the ankle application, especially for oils used to promote a restful night's sleep. Be sure to keep track of your applications so you can find the best solutions for your individual needs.

FEW Spots. FEW spots enable quick absorption through the largest pores on the body—feet, ears, and wrists. Known in Eastern medicine as the pipeline to the body, the soles of the feet have been used for centuries with reflexology to directly affect certain areas of the body. A reflexology chart will show you the corresponding areas of the body, and you can gently massage the oils where indicated for maximum benefit.

APPLICATION TECHNIQUES

Layering. Applying one oil at a time directly on top of another in a specific order is known as "layering." Apply one oil first, rub it in, wait a few seconds, and then apply the next. Repeat this process until all oils have been applied.

I don't necessarily recommend trying this without recommendation and guidance, but using several oils for the same issue can be extremely beneficial when layered. A trick for layering is to use what is called a "driver" oil last, such as Peppermint, since it will help the absorption of other oils.

Massage. Everyone can use a relaxing massage to de-stress or release tension, especially women after a long day. It is also a great way to boost the libido, as the sense of touch releases the feel-good hormone oxytocin. For therapeutic massage, I recommend using a 25 percent dilution, or one drop of oil for every three drops of carrier oil, or 25 drops in a teaspoon of carrier oil. Unless you are a certified massage therapist, I recommend starting with slow, gentle strokes and light pressure when using essential oils.

Compresses. Compresses allow the repulsion of oil and water to work to your benefit. After applying essential oils topically, add a wet, warm washcloth on top, allowing the water to push the oils in deeper. This will enhance the aromatherapeutic benefit of the oils. Cool-water compresses can help soothe away hot flashes, or ease the discomfort of muscle aches, swelling, sprains, or bruising.

Tee Shirt Tent. For aromatherapeutic benefit coupled with deep breathing, I recommend the "tee shirt tent." Place the essential oils down your décolletage, tuck your nose under your tee shirt, and practice your deep-breathing techniques. I recommend a few deep breaths in the tent, and then a few outside the tent, alternating until you feel relief. The oils will affect your bodily systems through direct absorption while allowing you to breathe in their benefits.

Baths. Bring on the nighttime self-care recipe and the soothing Epsom salt bath. Add ¼ cup of Epsom salts to warm bathwater first, swirling to dissolve, and then add three to six drops of essential oils. Without the salts, the essential oils will simply float on the surface of your bath. (And it doesn't hurt that Epsom salts are made from magnesium, which helps you go to sleep.) Do not soak for more than twenty minutes before rinsing off. Always hydrate well before and especially after your bath.

Internal Uses of Essential Oils

There is an ongoing debate in the aromatherapy community about ingesting essential oils, and I would only ever consider ingestion of pure high-quality therapeutic essential oils recommended for internal usage. Some oils are far more potent than others, and this is a decision you should make only after consulting a trusted health-care provider experienced in their use. Not all oils are recommended for internal consumption as a supplement, so do your homework. You will see that I do give guidelines for specific internal uses for oils throughout Part II, but those refer only to high-quality oils.

Personally, I love to add a drop of essential oils to my water infusions or green smoothies for enhanced flavor, but also because they support my immune system and hormonal balance. I often use herbal oils in my cooking as well, after checking that they are food-grade essential oils stamped with GRAS to ensure their certification.

It is not recommended to take essential oils internally when pregnant or breastfeeding unless you have been given the go-ahead by an aromatherapy expert or health-care practitioner.

Basic Essential Oil Supplies

Basic terminology in the essential-oil world can be confusing if you don't know the lingo. There are also certain supplies you will want to have on hand before beginning your journey. Following is a list of my must-have supplies, especially for the recipes in this book. The Resources (see page 351) will provide you with a link to my Getting Started with Essential Oils Checklist.

Carrier Oils

A carrier oil is an indispensable part of your essential-oil arsenal. It can be any kind of neutral vegetable, nut, or seed oil that blends well with essential oils to dilute them. Look for cold-pressed or expeller-pressed oils instead of solvent-extracted brands so you can avoid any added chemicals during the refining process. These are my favorite choices.

- **Organic Cold-Pressed Unrefined Coconut Oil.** At room temperature, coconut oil will be opaque white and semi-solid (like vegetable shortening), but becomes a clear liquid when slightly warmed. Unrefined oil retains the beachy smell that many of us love, but keep in mind that this scent will combine with whatever essential oil you use it with.

- **Organic Cold-Pressed Refined Coconut Oil.** The unscented version of the coconut oil described above. It works best to not compromise the aroma of the oils.
- **Fractionated Coconut Oil (FCO).** Always liquid at room temperature, FCO is my oil of choice for basic dilution and making rollerball bottles. I buy mine in a pump bottle for easy filling.
- **Jojoba Oil.** As it is closest to the natural sebum of our skin, I prefer jojoba oil when I'm making products that are applied to the face. Naturally greaseless and easily absorbable, jojoba oil has a long shelf life and is easily adaptable to a variety of skin-care products.
- **Sweet Almond Oil.** Another favorite for rollerball recipes, sweet almond oil is rich in vitamins B and E, but has a shorter shelf life than others. It should be avoided if you have any allergies to tree nuts.
- **Grapeseed Oil.** Slightly greenish, nutty-scented, and very light, grapeseed oil works well for massage oil blends.

Containers

While your essential oils should come in a tightly capped dark glass bottle fitted with an orifice reducer to control the flow of the oil and ensure it only comes out in drops, you might want a different-size container for your blends. These should also be dark glass with either an orifice reducer or a dropper top for ease of use.

Drams

Drams are tiny bottles used for sample sizes or on-the-go oils, and are usually 1- and 2-mL sizes. Most come with their own tiny orifice reducers that allow for smaller-sized drops. The reducers are easy to pop in but difficult to remove, so most people forgo refilling drams and just fill a new one. Some pipettes fit into the small holes for easy refilling. I tote around a collection of drams in my essential-oil keychain for all my on-the-go needs and especially when I'm traveling.

Dropper Tops

Dropper tops can easily replace the orifice reducer and cap on your essential-oil bottles and provide an easy way to measure out recipes. Be sure that you purchase dropper tops with glass tubes in the size meant to fit your size of bottles. Only one dropper top should be used per bottle, and you shouldn't switch them from one bottle to another. This is a personal preference, but I definitely think they come in handy for mixing rollerballs or filling drams.

Personal Inhalers

These little devices are small torpedo-shaped plastic containers meant to fit in the nostril. They diffuse your own personal blend of oils for easy inhalation. To use, simply uncap the lid, hold the tip up to a nostril, pinch the opposite one closed, and inhale. They are a discreet way to enhance your deep inhalation techniques.

To Make Your Own Personal Inhaler

- Personal inhaler
- Cotton wicks
- Glass dish or bowl
- Tweezers
- Essential oils of choice

Remove the cotton wick from the plug of the inhaler and lay it on a glass plate with a rim or in a bowl. Choose an essential oil or blend and have the bottles ready to go. The overall number of drops should be about 15, and simply add them directly on the wick. Tweezers can be used to move the wick around so that all essential oils are absorbed. Using your tweezers, pick up the wick and replace it into the plug and screw the cap back into the inhaler tube. Replace the cap tightly and you're ready to go.

Pipettes

Disposable plastic bulbs used for quick distribution of essential oils into other containers are known as pipettes. They are great if you don't want to spring for the more expensive dropper tops, as they are inexpensive. Be sure to use one pipette for each oil and do not mix them.

Rollerball Bottles

Usually found in 5 or 10 mL versions, rollerball bottles are glass cylinders fitted with a small plastic cap with a ball in it. These are my favorite containers to take my blends with me for easy application.

To apply the oils, you tip the bottle to moisten the ball, and then roll it directly on your skin. Many rollerball bottles are clear glass because they aren't expected to be stored for long, though dark glass versions are also an option. Keep an eye out for the oil in the bottle to become cloudy, however, which happens from frequent use due to dead skin cells that have rolled back into the bottle. When this happens, it's time to replace the oil.

To Make Your Own Rollerball Bottles

- Rollerball bottle
- Essential oils of choice
- Carrier oil of choice

Unscrew the cap and remove the rollerball top by popping it off with your thumb and forefinger. Set the glass bottle on a level surface and carefully fill with your rollerball blend recipe. Top off the rollerball with a carrier oil. When finished, replace the rollerball top by gently pushing it back into the glass bottle and tightly screwing the cap back on. Shake to combine the oils and apply.

Essential Oil Safety Tips

Honesty with Your Health-Care Provider

Honesty and openness with your trusted integrative health-care provider is the best policy. Since your provider will have your medical history, he or she may be able to properly advise you on using essential oils, especially if you have preexisting conditions or are already taking prescription medications. That said, many mainstream health-care professionals are not knowledgeable about essential oils and may discourage their use. A licensed naturopath, acupuncturist, herbalist, or aromatherapist will be able to give you expert advice.

Dilution

Dilution with a carrier oil not only increases the area of direct application but also helps to protect your skin from potential sensitivity. For adults, high-quality essential oils should always be diluted at least 25 percent, or 25 drops in a teaspoon of carrier oil. Some of the more skin-sensitive oils or phototoxic oils should be even further diluted (see pages 55 and 57 for details).

Oil Repels Water

The elementary school lesson that oil and water don't mix applies here as well. They naturally repel one another, which becomes an issue when you try to wash off an essential oil—it will only drive the oil deeper, intensifying your problem. Instead, you should always

dilute with a carrier oil to prevent further irritation or cross con-
tamination. Continue to dilute with a carrier oil every fifteen minutes until the irritation ceases.

These properties come in handy, however, when you want deeper
penetration of an oil. Then you can opt for a wet compress as described on page 49.

Patch-Testing

With any new essential oil, it is best to test for potential irritations first
before using it as planned in a recipe. Add one drop to one teaspoon
of a carrier oil and rub onto the bottom of your feet. Wait twenty-four
hours to see if there is any reaction, and, if not, then move on to another area and test again. Remember, if you *do* have a reaction, always
dilute it with a carrier oil rather than try to wash it off.

Phototoxicity/Photosensitivity

Phototoxic oils are those whose primary constituents react with
the sun by causing hyperpigmentation, blisters, or burns that can
potentially scar your body. An example of phototoxicity is using
lemon juice to lighten your hair in the summertime as an all-natural
alternative to expensive and toxic chemicals, but this same technique can be detrimental to the skin. I recommend not using these
particular oils on any exposed skin or when you will be in direct
exposure to sunlight or UV rays, especially in the summer or in hot
climates. Citrus oils are notoriously phototoxic, so use care when
exposing your skin to the application sites for at least 12 to 72 hours
post-application. Be extra careful when using some of the most phototoxic: Bergamot (the worst offender), Lemon, Lime, Grapefruit,
Wild Orange, or any cold-pressed citrus oil. Follow the guidelines
in this book when using these oils individually or with blends, but
generally use at least 1:4 dilution ratio, or 25 percent dilution, when
applying topically.

Potentially Phototoxic Essential Oils

Angelica	Coriander	Grapefruit	Orange
Anise	Cumin	Lemon	Tagetes
Bergamot	Dill	Lemon verbena	Tangerine
Bitter Orange	Fig Leaf Absolute	Lime	Wild Orange
Celery/Celery Leaf/Seed	Ginger	Mandarin Orange	Yuzu

Reactions

If you do have a reaction or a sensitivity to a particular essential oil, it is almost always because the oil has not been diluted enough. Sometimes there is an initial reaction only because the essential oil was too strong, so a higher level of dilution will still allow you to use it. For a reaction to occur, however, a plant protein must be present in the oil, though most proteins are removed during the distillation process.

If you know that you are allergic to a certain plant, flower, or spice, be extremely cautious when working with its essential oil, as you may have a reaction to its scent even if you don't touch the oil.

If there is any reaction, remember to *not* wash it off with water; dilute the area with more carrier oil over the next few hours until any irritation is gone. Always contact your health-care provider if you have any questions.

Skin-Sensitive Oils

Certain essential oils are skin-sensitive for everyone, even those without any allergies, and will *always* need to be diluted. They fall into two categories: hot or cool. Hot oils create a warming sensation that can easily cross into burning if they aren't diluted properly. Cooling oils create a cold, tingling sensation that can be very soothing, but can also become very uncomfortable to the skin.

Never apply hot or cool essential oils neat. Always follow the guidelines for dilution listed with each oil, and be careful not to cross-contaminate from one body part to another when using them. For example, don't touch any mucous membranes after applying these oils, especially your eyes or the inside of your mouth or nose.

As a general rule, I recommend at least a 10 percent dilution for each of the following oils, which means drops in a teaspoon of carrier oil.

Hot Oils

Cassia	Clove
Cinnamon	Hyssop
Cinnamon Bark	Oregano

Cool Oils

Camphor	Peppermint
Eucalyptus	Spearmint
Lemongrass	Thyme
Ocotea	Wintergreen

CHAPTER 3

The Top 15 Essential Oils for Hormones and the Value of Daily Usage

Essential oils can easily become a seamless part of your everyday routine once you give them a chance to work for you. Being consistent and persistent with daily usage is the key to rebalancing your body and creating the results that you desire.

Just be aware that the oils do not work the same way for each person, so trying different application methods and locations, the times of day you use them, and different combinations will serve you best in discovering your individual preferences.

Essential oils truly are gifts from nature for us to utilize to our benefit. Use these tips to make your essential oil journey an even more beneficial one:

The Top 15 Essential Oils
for Hormone Balance

For specific hormone benefits and other uses, see each chapter in Part II. Safety precautions are listed where applicable.

1. BASIL (*Ocimum basilicum*)

Primary Chemical Constituents: Linalool
Properties: Calming/Soothing
Safety Precautions

- Avoid if you are epileptic, pregnant, or breastfeeding.
- May affect blood clotting, so avoid if being treated for this disorder

2. BERGAMOT (*Citrus bergamia*)

Primary Chemical Constituents: Limonene, linalyl acetate
Properties: Uplifting/Energizing
Safety Precautions

- Extremely phototoxic—Avoid sunlight or UV rays for at least 72 hours after topical application.
- Avoid using if taking medication that increases sensitivity to sunlight.
- May lower blood sugar levels, so use caution if diabetic

The Top Five Must-Have Hormone Support Essential Oils for Women of Childbearing Age

Fennel	Thyme
Clary Sage	Ylang Ylang
Lavender	

What's in My Essential-Oil Kit

I never forget my essential-oil cases whenever I go out—they're basically an extension of who I am! Essential-oil cases are not only adorable but also practical; they're basically makeup bags with elasticized holders inside to keep the oils in place. (For where to get your own, see page 352.)

I use these oils all day long. They all smell wonderful and they're not just refreshing and delightful, but also targeted to all my needs. I'll always have different blends to ease tension, boost energy, manage cravings, and relax sore muscles. My Top Five single oils are always Wild Orange, Peppermint, Lavender, Clary Sage, and Neroli.

One of my favorite essential-oil blends is the Get It Done Rollerball Blend (page 107). It's a fantastic blend of Peppermint, Rosemary, Wild Orange, Basil, and Frankincense, the last probably one of the most powerful oils out there. Peppermint not only literally opens up the respiratory system but also increases energy and focus. It's like energy in a bottle and really gets me motivated. It's one of my secret weapons when I'm having one of those days, and even a go-go-go-getter like me can be dragging or procrastinating. One whiff and I'm right back on track.

3. CEDARWOOD (*Juniperus virginiana*)

Primary Chemical Constituents: α-cedrene, cedrol, thujopsene
Properties: Grounding/Balancing
Safety Precautions
• Avoid using during pregnancy.

4. CLARY SAGE (*Salvia sclarea*)

Primary Chemical Constituents: Linalyl acetate, linalool
Properties: Calming/Soothing

Safety Precautions

- Causes uterine contractions; avoid during pregnancy, but safe to use while in labor

5. GERANIUM (*Pelargonium graveolens*)

Primary Chemical Constituents: Citronellol, citronellyl formate, geraniol
Properties: Calming/Soothing

6. JASMINE ABSOLUTE (*Jasminum grandiflorum*)

Primary Chemical Constituents: Benzyl acetate, benzyl benzoate
Properties: Calming/Soothing
Safety Precautions
May cause mild allergic reactions owing to the benzyl acetate content

7. LAVENDER (*Lavandula angustifolia*)

Primary Chemical Constituents: Linalool, linalyl acetate
Properties: Calming/Soothing

8. LEMON (*Citrus limon*)

Primary Chemical Constituents: Limonene, β-Pinene, γ-terpinene
Properties: Uplifting/Energizing
Safety Precautions

- Phototoxic—dilute before topical application and avoid sunlight or UV rays for up to 12 hours after applying.

9. NEROLI (*Citrus x aurantium*)

Primary Chemical Constituents: Linalool, linalyl acetate, nerolidol
Properties: Calming/Soothing
Safety Precautions

- Avoid if you are taking a MAOI medication for depression or another issue.

10. PEPPERMINT (*Mentha piperita*)

Primary Chemical Constituents: Menthol, menthone, 1,8-cineole

Properties: Uplifting/Energizing

Safety Precautions

- Use caution if being treated for high blood pressure.
- Use caution if taking another medication for digestive health.
- Do not use within a 3-hour period of taking an iron supplement.
- Use caution if pregnant or breastfeeding, as it may reduce milk supply.
- Avoid using around children under 6 years of age due to high menthol content, which can slow breathing.

11. ROMAN CHAMOMILE (*Anthemis nobilis*)

Primary Chemical Constituents: 4-methylamyl angelate, iso-butyl angelate, isoamyl tiglate

Properties: Calming/Soothing

Safety Precautions

- Avoid using if you are pregnant or breastfeeding.

12. ROSEMARY (*Rosmarinus officinalis*)

Primary Chemical Constituents: 1,8-Cineole, α-Pinene, camphor

Properties: Renewing and Grounding/Balancing

Safety Precautions

- Avoid while pregnant or breastfeeding.
- Use caution if being treated for epilepsy, high blood pressure, or a bleeding disorder.

The Top 5 Must-Have Hormone Support Essential Oils for Perimenopausal/Menopausal Women

Clary Sage	Peppermint
Geranium	Rosemary
Lavender	

---

13. SANDALWOOD (HAWAIIAN) (*Santalum paniculatum*)

Primary Chemical Constituents: α-santalol, β-santalol, lanceol
Properties: Grounding/Balancing

14. THYME (*Thymus vulgaris*)

Primary Chemical Constituents: Thymol, para-cymene, γ-terpinene
Properties: Grounding/Balancing
Safety Precautions
- Dilute with a carrier oil owing to high thymol content prior to topical application.
- Avoid using if you have or are being treated for a blood-clotting disorder, as it may increase the risk of bleeding.

15. YLANG YLANG (*Cananga odorata*)

Primary Chemical Constituents: Germacrene, caryophyllene
Properties: Calming/Soothing

CHAPTER 4

The Importance of Creating Your Own Essential-Oil Rituals

In our modern world, we women frequently feel pressured to carry the weight of the world on our shoulders and strive to be all-things to everyone in that world. Love, compassion, understanding—these are the qualities expected of us as we bend over backward to care for and support our families, our friends, our co-workers, and just about everyone who crosses our path.

Except for one person—ourselves.

Whose permission are we waiting for to be compassionate to ourselves? It's time to shift our beliefs to include caring for ourselves along with everyone else.

Spending time focusing on yourself each day may seem like a selfish pursuit, but I can assure you it is precisely the opposite. We can't help others find success if we aren't in top condition ourselves. And when we constantly put others' needs above our own, when we cannot find it in ourselves to say no, when we tell ourselves we can be fueled by stress, we neglect to nurture our own needs.

We are the ones who suffer the consequences.

Health issues, hormonal imbalance, mood swings, sleep issues, unhealthy weight gain, and many more symptoms crop up, one by one. But we even tend to ignore *those* symptoms in favor of pushing forward and maintaining our outward appearance of being in complete control.

Don't let yourself get to that breaking point. Don't let your foundations crumble until you become unrecognizable even to yourself.

You matter. Your life matters. Your emotional health matters. Your hormonal balance matters. Your *everything* matters.

You deserve to treat yourself with the same love and compassion that you dole out to the world. Self-care rituals with essential oils enable you to find yourself amid the chaos of everyday life, and truly love yourself in the skin you're in. Rebalancing, refocusing, and reflecting each day will help you to stay in tune with your body, mind, and soul.

What Are Self-Care Rituals?

Every aspect of life is punctuated by ritual, from the way you get out of bed to the way you do the dishes, from seasonal events to holiday traditions, from the method you use to eat your food to the way you navigate the grocery store. Whether you realize it or not, your daily routine is full of ritualistic behavior unique to you.

The rituals featured in this book are all about creating a routine that will boost and balance your body and mind to bring balance and joy to your life. Each of us will have to determine the rituals that work best for us, and none of us will go about them quite the same way. The support of essential oils is the one consistent factor. All the chapters in Part II contain self-care rituals that you can immediately use to boost your energy and enhance your world.

You Deserve It!

The reason behind the rituals is simple: *You deserve them.*

The feeling that we are not deserving of self-care, of the best of what life has to offer, is a major issue that plagues us as women in our society now. I know exactly what they're saying, because I didn't grow up with my own worth being affirmed to me. I adapted

---

The Love & Joy List

One of the things I ask women to do all the time is to create a twenty-item Love & Joy List on a piece of lined paper. Each item you add to that list is something that brings you love and joy. The paper is divided into two groups; on the left side, you write down ten things that cost money, and on the right, ten things that are free. For example, my list would include flowers, essential oils, and massages on the left, and quality time with my hubby, reading a good novel, walking on the beach, and hiking on the right.

Some women find this activity a little uncomfortable at first because they've never been asked what they love or what brings them joy. When they finally finish their lists, their faces beam; they realize they can still find love and joy in their lives. It's a great double-dose of self care and acknowledgment of self-worth.

Identifying your twenty items and writing them down reinforces the notion of *your* doing things for *you*. Then, you can take a good, hard look at the list and figure out how to create self-care rituals unique to your needs and desires to ensure that love and joy become a daily part of your life. I encourage you to create your own list and use it to tweak the rituals in this book to be perfect for you!

---

to this lapse of support by throwing myself headfirst into life, thinking that if I wasn't doing the work—*more* work, in fact, than anyone had the right to ask of me—then I was a failure.

I didn't just wake up one day and not be able to lift my head up off the pillow—it took *years* to get to that point, along with lots of signs and symptoms I ignored. But the essential-oil component is what truly turned my world around.

Once I discovered the power of essential oils, I realized that they didn't have to be used only in times of great need. Over a decade ago, I created several rituals, easy to implement every day, that now serve as a foundational part of my life. I encourage you to examine these rituals closely and work to incorporate them into your life, too. I don't want to fall back into the danger zone of my old bad habits, and my rituals keep me proactively in charge. Though I had to start purposefully incorporating them into my daily routine, they are now deeply ingrained habits.

Before You Start Your Rituals

Start Slow. Jumping right in by trying to incorporate every ritual that you love will only create more stress than the calm and self-love you are seeking. Baby steps will prevent you from slipping into ritual overwhelm.

Choose One Ritual. Start with the one ritual that appeals to you the most. Many women gravitate toward an evening ritual, as this enables them to unwind at the end of the day and de-stress from life's chaotic pace. Work that ritual into your day, and when you can't imagine *not* doing it, move on to the next one.

Prep in Advance. Be sure to have your essential oils, recipes, and directions at hand so you don't become overwhelmed by the routine. Get everything that you need ready to go and then let yourself fall into the ritual. Eventually, it will become second-nature to you, but give yourself an advantage by having your materials ready so you don't have to break the routine to get up and find something.

Essential Oils to Go. Always have your essential oils with you. When I'm at work, my little stash is near me on my desk, always within reach. I have an essential-oils keychain in my purse for on-the-go needs, and you know my rollerball clutch travels with me in my purse. Find a way to take your oils with you so that rituals can be adaptable when you need them the most.

Joy! Whatever you choose as your personal rituals, they should all leave you resonating with joy. This should not be a stressful or uncomfortable experience for you. If you don't find joy in it, then don't do it.

A Glimpse into My World— My Daily Rituals

Because I want you to feel supported and know that you are not alone, I want to share the rituals that work best for me. Remember that the suggestions I give as self-care rituals are just that—it's up to you to work your own positivity into them to make them your own. Creating your own routine should bring you the joy, love, and peace that mine bring me!

The Morning Ritual: Starting Your Day Right and Scheduling Your Wellness

One of my favorite quotes is from Louise Hay: "How you start your day is how you live your day. How you live your day is how you live your life."

Starting your morning with positive self-care rituals can powerfully influence your entire day. You will establish and gain clarity and purpose, and set your intentions and tone so that you accomplish your goals. Morning rituals can be anything you desire—just be sure that you take some quality time for yourself and don't allow the ritual to be interspersed between your other tasks, such as getting the kids ready for school. You are giving yourself the time to center yourself and focus on *you*, which will make everyone's morning go more smoothly.

Women who struggle with their intentions often tell me that they *can't* do this or that, but usually these are red flags signaling that they are avoiding something, or associated with fear. Self-care rituals may help you to discover your inner demons and learn to love yourself for who you truly are. Use your morning ritual to help you to prioritize your intentions for the day and support those beliefs with essential oils to help you take on the tasks ahead.

These are the self-care rituals I use to start my day each morning. They only take me twenty to thirty minutes and are absolutely worth it.

Shower Ritual: I include my Invigorating Morning Bliss Shower Spray (page 108) to get myself in the game for the rest of the day.

Essential Oil Ritual: Diffusing Peppermint and Wild Orange in the morning is my go-to for an instant energy boost while I prep my green smoothie. Depending on my mood, I might grab my Superwoman Rollerball Blend (page 300) and apply it to my wrists and other pulse points to hone my femininity and prepare for my upcoming tasks.

Playlist Ritual: Though music plays a huge role in my everyday life, I always put on one of my playlists as soon as I'm out of the shower and getting ready. I love soul music, especially Stevie Wonder, Aretha Franklin, and Earth Wind and Fire, and hearing any of their songs always puts me in a really great place.

Journal Ritual: My all-time-favorite journal is called *Speed Dial the Universe*, a fantastic tool laid out with different sections. All I have to do is fill in the blanks. Writing everything down helps me to set my intentions for the day, and it's probably one of the most game-changing things that I do for myself. Because I'm driven by what I'm writing, I find these moments help me find extreme clarity in tough situations or just approaching my tasks. It gives me a path to follow, because I can always go back to any given day in my journal to discover where I was and what I was thinking. My journal allows me to focus on what I'm doing for *me*. Believe it or not, I've been faithfully writing in my journals for ten years, and it's my must-do.

To-Do Sanity List Ritual: I love lists! They really help me give structure to and sort out my tasks for the day, and it is deeply satisfying to cross each item off the list once I get it done. When I know I have a lot to do, I write down my big-action to-do's early in the morning in my journal. Once I write them down, they're inked in my memory and become must-do's for the day. For reinforcement, I use my Get It Done Rollerball Blend (page 107)—the oils that I know will fire me up.

Schedule Your Success Ritual: I make purposeful time in my day by scheduling time for myself. This helps me include the rituals, meals, and so on. I schedule everything! I know lots of women like me who admit, if it's not on the calendar, it won't get done or is forgotten.

Inspiration Ritual: One of my favorite rituals is inhaling Frankincense essential oil for inspiration, focus, and concentration, then spending a few minutes writing in my gratitude journal.

Strengthening Daytime Rituals for Sustained Energy

Although your daytime rituals can be as varied as your schedule, there are some that I do no matter what time of day it is or where I am.

Breathe-on-the-Hour Ritual: So simple, yet so effective, especially at keeping those cortisol levels on an even keel and de-stressing your life. Set your cellphone's alarm to ring every hour of the day. When the phone sounds, take a minute or two to inhale whatever essential oil you need, practicing deep-breathing techniques, and using that moment to pause.

Nature Nurtures Ritual: Being out in nature truly brings me joy, and I can't imagine my life without those long walks and hikes. Not only is walking an ideal way for you to get your body moving but also breathing in the fresh air and being outside can bring a new sense of joy to your day.

The Evening Ritual to End Your Day Right

Your evening ritual is just as important as your morning ritual. I hope you will do this one, as it is one of the most empowering rituals you can add to your life.

Mirror Ritual: Look in the mirror and say some of your positive affirmations. You know you are a strong, capable, and sexy woman. Tell yourself this until you believe it. *Champion your successes* by affirming your accomplishments or whatever means the most in your world. *Acknowledge your strengths;* I often say, "I'm an incredible healer. I serve thousands of people with grace and energy. I forgive myself. I'm an amazing wife." (I have to say that a lot!) *Show Yourself Some Love.* Finish your mirror ritual by saying "I love you!" I often forget that one because I'm so hard on myself (I'm sure you know the feeling!). It might feel silly at first, but supporting yourself with an "I Love You" really does boost your sense of self-worth. Trust me—this is going to make you feel amazing! It's the perfect way to end your day on a high note.

Incorporating the power of essential oils was game-changing for my rituals. Their immediate effect afforded me long-lasting resolution of many issues I had been facing. From something as simple as energizing my mind in the morning to the more complicated nuances of hormonal balance, essential oils have been the bridge that kept me from toppling headfirst into the gap. You'll see that transforming your life with these rituals will give you not only power but also balance and comfort—they're an entirely new way to supercharge and enhance your day.

PART II

Using Essential Oils to Address Your Hormonal Symptoms

CHAPTER 5

Stress

As a strong, ambitious, *d-r-i-v-e-n* woman, I know what it means to be everything to everyone. I lived it. I breathed it. I defined myself by my ability to do just that. Until I couldn't anymore. I had allowed myself to believe a lie for years and years.

What was the lie? *That I was fueled by stress.*

I said it to people who commented about how driven I was. I said it to my professors who thought I was taking on too much. I said it to my bosses, who may or may not have treated me differently because I was a female in a male-driven society. I said it to myself whenever I noticed a symptom that had never appeared before—right before I pushed it back down inside me and pushed forward into what I thought was success.

By the time I hit my mid-twenties, the symptoms became more than I could ignore, more than I could manage, and I began to feel broken. I was a hot mess! But guess what I did? Pushed myself even harder and continued the "I am fueled by stress" mantra as if it were a *good* thing.

As I approached the big 3-0, I felt more like an old lady than the vibrant and successful woman I appeared to others. But it was getting harder and harder to hide from the symptoms that plagued me on a daily, hourly, minute-by-minute basis. Exhausted, plagued by migraines, and incapable of putting on my game face and carrying on, I slowly began to realize the self-sabotage I had created—but this was *not* who I was. The stress that ruled my life needed to leave; I had so much more to give. I was worthy and deserving of the kind of self care that I so easily gave to my patients, yet somehow couldn't give to myself. I finally admitted to the giant lie that for so long had been destroying me.

Guess what happened? The more care I took of myself, the more capable I became as a healer, a doctor, a wife, and a woman.

How did I lasso that stress and regain control of my life? It was not easy. It was a slow process of taking responsibility, being mindful of those stressful moments, and using my essential oils to reach the healthy, vivacious woman I knew I could be.

Looking back now, I realize that moment was my epiphany. By admitting that I had allowed myself to be negatively fueled by stress, that I had allowed that stress to slowly destroy me, I realized that the *stress* was the problem and *not* me. I sought out professional help, made foundational lifestyle changes, harnessed the power of essential oils, and found myself in the process.

Because I know what it feels like to be dominated by stress, I began questioning my patients. Every one of them admitted to being stressed. They also had fed the lie that they could work through it, manage it, and survive despite it. "Stressed?" they'd say with a laugh. "Yes, I'm stressed, but who isn't? I probably have too much on my plate and, yes, I'm tired all the time—but if I don't do it, who will? My family comes first, so I just keep on doing what I'm doing!"

And then I had to break the bad news. I'd tell them how, in ten years, they wouldn't be able to take care of their family, because the symptoms they were experiencing now were just the tip of the iceberg. Stress was going to eat away at their very foundation until they couldn't care for themselves, let alone their families.

Tears would fill their eyes. They weren't happy. They were struggling and suffering. They didn't feel appreciated, either by their husbands or partners, or their family, or their work. They thought life was supposed to be lived through obligation, which wore them down. They felt broken, just as I had.

Even worse, many of these women, especially those close to or over fifty, had given up. They accepted their current state of being as *their* normal—and had been told that normal for their age meant *hormonal*, that they had to brace themselves for "the change"—the weight gain, low libido, hot flashes, brain fog, exhaustion. Basically, they had to prepare for the end.

It was utterly heartbreaking. The lies they were told, the supposed truths of nature that they believed—it doesn't have to be this way.

The Why *Behind Stress*

To understand the effects of stress, you need to understand how the body functions when stress enters its world. The human body is designed to respond in specific ways to acute stress, or short-term stressors, in order to protect itself in favor of survival. Hormones rush in, shutting down unnecessary systems, and the body shifts into "fight-or-flight" mode to keep danger at bay and itself alive. When the stress response is used properly, it helps the body stay safe by kicking us into action. Many of us love the slight adrenaline rush that this provides! Then, once the stress has been managed, the body's systems return to normal and rebalances.

The problem is that our twenty-first-century world doesn't function the way life did in prehistoric times. Saber-toothed tigers and hunting for food once provided that short-term stress, but now we become stressed at something as simple as a television commercial reminding us we haven't planned for retirement. Our personalities play into this conundrum as well; introverts may worry and overthink situations, while extroverts can feel isolated by spending too much time alone. This leads our bodies into a pattern known as *episodic acute stress,* which keeps our bodies constantly on guard.

Regardless of the stressor or trigger, acute stress causes our bodies to divert blood flow from our digestive and reproductive systems and to redirect it to our extremities in preparation for a full-on battle. Blood pressure and heart rate increase, respiration kicks into high drive, and we are primed for battle. But then, the battle is meant to be over so our bodies can calm down, rebalance, and get back to normal. If they don't, this develops into a long-term, chronic stress disaster.

Ignoring stress is *the biggest trigger* for your hormonal symptoms because it affects so many different bodily functions, down to the cellular level. The mitochondria in our cells serve as powerhouses that allow our bodies to function, affecting everything from cell metabolism to hormone production, immune system to emotional response, and more. The primary task of the mitochondria is to convert the food we eat into ATP (adenosine triphosphate), our energy storage system. During this process, however, normal oxidative stress is created; if we don't produce enough, our bodies can become susceptible to attack, such as infections, illnesses, and trauma. But the bigger problem occurs when chronic stress overloads our bodies with even more oxidative stress. This causes cell death. And when cells die, our bodies age.

We are complicating our body chemistry like we've never done before—instituting a real crisis. Let's take a look at physical, mental/emotional, and chemical/toxic stress.

Physical Stress

Basic Definition: Any form of stress that affects your physical body. When you overload your body with too many expectations and too much to do, and then prevent its circadian rhythm from allowing it to recuperate during sleep, coupled with poor nutrition that cannot properly provide the energy your body needs as fuel, you're dealing with physical stress. It can also be affected by the effects of illness, especially chronic illness, which weakens your body's ability to complete the tasks required of it.

Symptoms: Absent libido, aches and pains, acne, anxiety, appetite changes, chest pain, decreased energy, dizziness, dry mouth, fatigue, frequent illness (colds, cold sores, infections), gastrointestinal distress, hair loss, headaches/migraines, heart palpitations, inability to focus, increased heart rate, insomnia, muscle tension, muscle spasms, panic attacks, rashes, sweating without exertion, teeth grinding or jaw clenching, tics or nervous habits, tinnitus, tremors, weight gain or loss, and more.

Emotional/Mental Stress

Basic Definition: Any form of stress that affects your mood or mental state. Chronic worry and feeling overwhelmed, without the ability to relax, lead to emotional and mental stress, as do emotionally taxing or devastating events, such as losing a job, bankruptcy, an accident or injury, or the loss of a loved one.

Symptoms: Agitation, antisocial behavior, anger, anxiety, confusion, depression, edginess, emotional outbursts, guilt, forgetfulness, frustration, hostility, insomnia, irritability, isolation, loneliness, low self-esteem, mental chatter, nervousness, overreaction to situations, obsessive or compulsive behavior, overwhelm, restlessness, suicidal thoughts, tension, feelings of worthlessness, and more.

In its most recent annual "Stress in America" report, the American Psychological Association said that 80 percent of Americans reported experiencing at least one symptom associated with stress in a month's period, with the most common being headache, feelings of being overwhelmed, nervousness and anxiety, or depression. They acknowledge the toll physical and emotional stress can have on our everyday health. And who reported the highest levels of stress? *Women.*

But you *are* in control! You *can* make choices to de-stress your life and use essential oils to create ease and grace.

The Hormones for Stress

Adrenaline and Cortisol

Your body's cortisol levels are meant to fluctuate throughout the day. Normally, they rise throughout the night, peak in the morning hours, then lower again into the evening hours. This is known as diurnal rhythm, and it helps the body to maintain its natural balance. Cortisol is vital for cognitive function, metabolic balance, and many other processes.

When stressors come into play, the body springs into action. As you know, our adrenal glands are the primary players in stress regulation. *Adrenaline* (epinephrine) is released as soon as any kind of stressful situation arises, automatically forcing our bodies into the fight-or-flight response. Our heart rate and blood pressure increase and our energy boosts in favor of winning the impending battle. *Cortisol* comes next, boosting glucose in the bloodstream to produce energy for the fight. Since the adrenal glands can't distinguish what triggered your stress, they're going to pump out cortisol, no matter what. Add chronic levels of stress to this equation and you have a constant cycle of adrenal activation, with elevated stress hormones. Hello, HPA axis dysregulation.

Some of the more common symptoms of HPA axis deregulation from high cortisol levels include feeling overwhelmed owing to unmanaged stress, tired-but-wired fatigue, skin issues, insomnia, unexplainable mood swings, weight gain, frequent bouts of illness, irregular menstrual cycles, and libido issues, among others. Eventually this may lead to serious medical issues, such as Cushing's syndrome (chronic and excess levels of cortisol in the bloodstream).

T3 and T4

When the body experiences stress, it decreases thyroid function in favor of conserving energy for whatever fight may be ahead. In a normal acute stress situation, this is a good thing, as the body needs to do this for fight-or-flight or healing. The problem surfaces when the body constantly suppresses thyroid function owing to *chronic* stress, affecting every system on the HPA axis.

Remember that, normally, T4 converts to T3, and a small bit gets converted into Reverse T3 to keep your system balanced. Increased stress triggers TSH (Thyroid-Stimulating Hormone) to produce even less free T3 and an increased amount of Reverse T3, causing your metabolism to slow down to preserve energy—but too much Reverse T3 also blocks thyroid-hormone receptors. The other most significant indirect effect the adrenals have on thyroid function is via their influence on blood sugar. High or low cortisol can cause hypoglycemia, hyperglycemia, or both. Blood sugar imbalances cause hypothyroid symptoms if left unchecked.

Cortisol also disrupts the delicate balance of the HPT axis (hypothalamic-pituitary-thyroid), which relies on it as well as on melatonin to keep thyroid levels even. Sadly, many practitioners don't check for the Reverse T3 levels, leaving you dealing with symptoms with no end in sight.

Insulin

When your body kicks into the fight-or-flight response, the liver also produces more glucose to give you the energy you need. Whatever isn't used should be reabsorbed by the body, but those more at risk for Type 2 diabetes and stress-induced hyperglycemia will lose the ability to respond to insulin and eventually become insulin resistant. Studies reported by the National Institutes of Health have shown that repeated insulin spikes, commonly seen with insulin resistance, increase the destruction of the thyroid gland in people with autoimmune thyroid disease.

Estrogen and Progesterone

Chronic stress leads to anovulation, amenorrhea, and other potential menstrual issues and irregularities. And when menopause approaches, hormone levels begin to fluctuate and decline, and the symptoms that arise from neglected foundational systems can cause even more stress on your body. Dealing with the aging process often triggers emotional stress as well.

Emotional Triggers for Stress

Identifying what plagues you emotionally and learning to deal with it proactively can be the best step in managing your personal stress levels. We all have experienced the intense symptoms of emotional stress, and this is where I rely a lot on my intuition—that inner voice that directs me, that gut feeling that stops me in my tracks, that twinge I get when something sends up a red flag. Learning to notice those signs rather than ignore them will be the key to beginning to manage your stress rather than allowing it to manage *you*.

I know stress has gotten the best of me when I start sweating the small stuff, or when the tiniest thing sets me into a whirlwind of worry. What I'm upset about may have nothing to do with the actual problem, but it ends up being the last straw. Like the time my husband decided to buy a new kind of almond milk. We try new foods all the time and usually this piques my curiosity, but on that particular day I was completely overwhelmed and stressed out. Instead of welcoming his spontaneity, I bit the poor man's head off. Luckily, he knew how stressed I was and managed to calm me down by simply going to the essential-oils cabinet and handing me my Tense-Away Rollerball Blend (page 89), then slowly backing away. I knew by his reaction that mine had been way more than I intended, but it made me sit down and take a look at why I had overreacted to almond milk!

Take the time to reflect, and ask yourself the following questions:

- What triggers my stress or my emotional outbursts?
- What stress can I manage?

- What stress bothers me to where I can't move on from it?
- What can I change in my life to manage the stress better?
- What am I unable to change, and what will I do to cope?

Allow yourself to be *pro*active rather than *re*active. Employ self-care rituals and essential oils to help you make the move from stress to chill. Reset your lifestyle by paying attention to the foundational lifestyle changes discussed in Chapter 1. And give yourself the gift of self-love by making time for yourself.

How to Calm Stress with Essential Oils

Finding the calm amid the chaos of life and the never-ending stressors can be achieved one drop at a time with these preferred essential oils.

Preferred Essential Oils

BERGAMOT (*Citrus bergamia*)
- Dissolves anxious feelings while uplifting the emotions
- Cleanses and purifies the mind and body
- Lowers stress levels

Aromatic Use
- Diffuse during times of intense stress to enhance calm.
- Diffuse to promote self-confidence while developing a sense of inner peace and calm.

Topical Use
- Apply as a massage oil diluted with your favorite carrier oil.
- Make your own face mask with organic Greek yogurt and organic raw honey.
- Massage into body while taking a shower.

- To promote a restful night's sleep, dilute and apply to the bottoms of feet before bedtime.

WARNING: Avoid direct exposure to sunlight or UV rays after topical use of Bergamot as it is phototoxic.

CEDARWOOD (*Juniperus virginiana*)

- Soothes and grounds the mind and body to promote vitality and relaxation
- Aids in emotional balance and overall wellness
- Allows the body to find a natural calm and confidence

Aromatic Use

- Diffuse 2–4 drops.
- Diffuse 2 drops with 2 drops Lavender.

Topical Use

- Massage 1–3 drops with 1 teaspoon of carrier oil onto chest during workouts or meditation/prayer.
- In moments of severe stress or panic, massage into pulse points.

WARNING: Not recommended for internal usage.

CLARY SAGE (*Salvia sclarea*)

- Provides calm and relaxation to the mind and body
- Alleviates muscle tension and cramping while promoting relaxation
- Supports a restful night's sleep by calming mental chatter and enhancing overall calm

Aromatic Use

- Diffuse 3–4 drops.
- Add 1–2 drops to pillows or bedclothes.

Topical Use

- Massage 1–3 drops with 1 teaspoon of carrier oil into the abdomen.
- Apply 1–2 drops with your favorite carrier oil onto your soles or over pulse points.
- Add 2–3 drops to an Epsom salts bath or your favorite all-natural body wash.

FRANKINCENSE (*Boswellia carterii, B. frereana,* and *B. sacra*)

- Promotes feelings of relaxation and calm
- Supports bodily systems (immune, nervous, digestive) and cellular function when taken internally

Aromatic Use

- Diffuse 3–4 drops.
- Add 1 drop rubbed in the palms and inhale deeply.
- Add 20 drops Frankincense, 20 drops Bergamot, and 20 drops Lavender to a 2-ounce glass spray bottle, and fill the rest with distilled water or witch hazel. Shake and spritz around the house for a DIY room refresher.

Topical Use

- Apply 1–2 drops with your favorite carrier oil to your soles.
- Add to your favorite moisturizer.

LAVENDER (*Lavandula angustifolia*)

- Soothes the mind and body to promote overall calm
- Supports the body in a restful night's sleep
- Melts away tension and anxiety

Aromatic Use

- Add 1–2 drops to bedclothes and pillows.
- Diffuse 3–4 drops before bed.

Topical Use

- Dab on pulse points.
- Apply 1–2 drops with your favorite carrier oil to your soles before bedtime.
- Add 2–3 drops to an Epsom salts bath or add to your favorite all-natural body wash.

WILD ORANGE (*Citrus sinensis*)

- Uplifts and energizes the mind and body
- Eases digestive discomfort
- Purifies and stimulates the body's system, especially the immune system

Aromatic Use
- Add 1–2 drops to a diffuser.
- Add 1 drop to your palm with 1 drop each of Peppermint and Frankincense and your favorite carrier oil, rub together, and inhale deeply.

Topical Use
- Apply the Wild Orange–Peppermint–Frankincense blend from above to the back of your neck.
- Add to your body wash.
- Dilute with a carrier oil and apply to your abdomen with Peppermint.

WARNING: Avoid direct exposure to sunlight or UV rays after topical use of Wild Orange, as it is phototoxic.

Debra's Story

Debra was thirty-nine years old when she came to me, concerned with multiple symptoms that seemed to have shown up suddenly. She had gained almost eleven pounds over the course of three months, despite running three miles four or five times a week. She also found herself having a difficult time falling asleep at night owing to anxiousness, and was encountering more stress at her job as an analyst because of recent layoffs. Drinking more iced coffee in the afternoon than normal, she tried to compensate for her lack of sleep, but instead found herself forgetting little things, like where she placed her keys.

Hormone testing showed that Debra was suffering from chronic stress, high cortisol levels, and higher than normal estrogen levels. **My recommendations were as follows:**

- For afternoon slumps, a combination of Spearmint and Wild Orange essential oils for focus.
- Crave-Control Rollerball Blend (page 147) after dinner to avoid late-night cravings.
- For sleep, Deep Relaxation Diffuser Blend (page 127) in a diffuser 2 hours before bed. Lavender and Vetiver on her neck and feet before going to bed.
- Gratitude journal each morning with Wild Orange essential oil.
- Short-burst interval exercises to ramp up her metabolism and burn more fat three times a week. Yoga twice a week for stress reduction.
- Replace coffee with matcha green tea. The L-theanine in green tea reduces stress without causing sedation.
- More green leafy vegetables at each meal to support healthy estrogen metabolism.
- Supplements: a multivitamin, 300 mg magnesium glycinate, 500 mg of ashwagandha, Tulsi tea in the morning, and 2000 mg of omega-3 fatty acids to lower stress levels and increase lean body mass.

Within three weeks, Debra experienced more energy, especially in the middle of the day. She was sleeping seven or more hours each night. She lost six pounds and felt less stressed at work, especially after taking five-minute breaks with her **Stress Relief Rollerball Blend** (page 89). Her late-night cravings were gone and her memory felt restored. When I asked how her energy levels were, she replied, "I can't imagine my life without these wonderful oils! I love incorporating them into my day, especially while I am working. I feel confident with the tools I have to support my body."

Essential Oil Blends

Aromatic Diffuser Blends

Reset and Restore Diffuser Blend

2 drops Cedarwood essential oil
2 drops Wild Orange essential oil
1 drop Ylang Ylang essential oil

Chillax Diffuser Blend

3 drops Lavender essential oil
2 drops Clary Sage essential oil
2 drops Cedarwood essential oil

Ground and Calm Diffuser Blend

2 drops Bergamot essential oil
2 drops Frankincense essential oil
2 drops Lavender essential oil

Aromatic Personal Inhaler Blends

Bounce Back Inhaler Blend

4 drops Bergamot essential oil
4 drops Ylang Ylang essential oil
4 drops Lavender essential oil
3 drops Wild Orange essential oil

Zen Inhaler Blend

4 drops Clary Sage essential oil
4 drops Wild Orange essential oil
4 drops Frankincense essential oil
3 drops Cedarwood essential oil

Focus and Uplift Inhaler Blend

4 drops Rosemary essential oil

3 drops Bergamot essential oil

3 drops Wild Orange essential oil

2 drops Peppermint essential oil

1 drop Frankincense essential oil

Aromatic Room and Body Spray

De-Stress Spritz

10 drops Wild Orange essential oil

8 drops Lavender essential oil

5 drops Clary Sage essential oil

1½ ounces distilled water

Add essential oils to a 2-ounce glass spray bottle and top off with water. Cap the bottle and shake to combine. Spritz in the air or on your body.

Topical Rollerball Blends

Stress Relief Rollerball Blend

12 drops Lavender essential oil

9 drops Frankincense essential oil

9 drops Tangerine essential oil

Carrier oil of choice

Add essential oils to a 10 mL glass rollerball bottle and top off with carrier oil of your choice. Replace the rollerball top and cap, and shake gently to combine. Apply blend to your soles, back of neck, or palms.

Tense-Away Rollerball Blend

10 drops Lavender essential oil

10 drops Clary Sage essential oil

10 drops Peppermint essential oil

Carrier oil of choice

Add essential oils to a 10 mL glass rollerball bottle and top off with carrier oil of choice. Replace the rollerball top and cap, and shake gently to combine. Roll on wrists, ankles, back of neck, and on any tense areas, then massage in. Deeply inhale the aroma from your wrists whenever tension creeps back in.

Motivate and Recharge Rollerball Blend

10 drops Wild Orange essential oil
10 drops Peppermint essential oil
7 drops Ylang Ylang essential oil
3 drops Basil essential oil
Carrier oil of choice

Add essential oils to a 10 mL glass rollerball bottle and top off with carrier oil of choice. Replace the rollerball top and cap, and shake gently to combine. Roll on wrists, behind ears, and back of neck. Deeply inhale the aroma from your wrists whenever you need a quick recharge.

Self-Care Rituals for Stress

Daily self-care stress-busting rituals train your mind and body to focus on itself, to find the calm in the storm, and to refocus and recharge during potential chaos. Allow yourself the time to become familiar with your favorite options and begin to incorporate them into your daily stress-relieving regimen. But to begin, know that the number one priority is you: *you* scheduling a permanent appointment with *yourself.*

Self-care time must be nonnegotiable. Even if you only start with a few minutes every day, your mind and body need that time to reclaim their focus and vitality. It's time that will allow you to pause life and escape from the stress. So, go read a book, laugh at cat videos, soak in nature on a walk or hike, relax and unwind in the bath, try a new recipe—whatever makes you smile. Just be sure to do something you love, completely uninterrupted.

Power of Pause Ritual

Incorporate the pause ritual into your daily deep-breathing exercises and couple it with a diffuser blend or personal inhaler for super-charged results. Simply breathe in deeply by expanding your diaphragm, allowing your belly to push out, and then pause for five seconds at the top of that inhale. Then exhale slowly, letting your belly button pull in toward your spine, and at the pit, pause and simply be in that moment. Allow yourself to repeat five to ten times for a cortisol-lowering calm, anywhere you need it. Meditation and prayer greatly benefit from these suspended pauses, and you can train yourself to hold them longer as you get better at the process.

Laugh It Off Ritual

Many people say that laughter is the best medicine, and according to the Mayo Clinic, they are correct. Laughing depresses your stress responses and cortisol levels, allowing more oxygen in to enhance relaxation. Find something that makes you belly-laugh and allow yourself to unwind by relishing in humor.

Get a Move On Ritual

Exercise, as you will see in Chapter 6, amps up your heart health, supports your brain, and helps to lower tension and cortisol levels. The key is to allow it to be a stress reliever instead of a stress inducer. Exercise should be a way for you to release the weight of the world, so find something that you really love. Take a dance class or just have a dance party in your kitchen, try some hot yoga, or strap on gloves and box away your pent-up tension, or hike a mountain, or simply take a walk.

Meditate and Breathe Ritual

Mind–body exercises such as yoga or tai chi gently work your body while they calm the mind. I love guided meditation apps that gently lead me through the process of meditation and/or deep breathing. Add a calming blend to your diffuser or rollerball a Zen-band on your wrists and spend some self-care time in reflection and pause. I also recommend GPS for the Soul, an app that measures your HRV (heart rate variability)—the interval between each heartbeat as an indicator of resilience—with the camera on your phone. This revolutionary heart-math technology lowers your cortisol and DHEA levels by training your mind to eliminate negative thought patterns.

Massage Ritual

A therapeutic massage lowers cortisol and promotes deep relaxation, as well as the release of the brain chemicals dopamine and serotonin—which is one of the reasons why you feel so good afterward. Supporting therapeutic massage with essential oils will enhance the powerful effect.

Stress-Busting Playlist Ritual

Music, like laughter, influences stress levels depending on what you listen to. Loud, abrasive music can set your teeth on edge, but soothing, rhythmic music—such as classical, New Age, or even nature sounds—clicks your mind out of its stress while reducing anxiety. Smart doctors and dentists offer their patients headphones and a choice of music to calm frayed nerves before medical procedures.

Minimize stress by creating your own magic and comforting playlist for your daily routine. Very quickly, your body will hear the soothing tunes and instantly start to relax. Many mamas know this secret already, as they calm their babies with lullabies, many of whom learned the melodies while still in the womb.

Enjoy Nature Ritual

One of the best stress-busting rituals I do for myself is take a hike—literally! Being outside in the fresh air recharges, rejuvenates, and gives me a chance to decompress, even if it's only for twenty minutes. No matter how difficult my day has been or what tasks are awaiting me when I get home, nature *always* reduces my stress and gives me a chance to clear my head. Find some time to reconnect with nature, allow the sun to recharge your vitamin D, and reflect on the wonder of the world in which we live.

CHAPTER 6

Energy and Fatigue

In high school, I was the girl who volunteered for every extracurricular activity while maintaining her A average; who set her sights on becoming valedictorian and didn't stop until she achieved it. I was determined to be everything for everyone. I gave off a persona of an indefatigable superwoman even at the age of seventeen. Everyone bought it.

A decade later, everyone who met me always said that I had incredible energy. They continued to buy the lie I was selling. So did I. Until I crashed with a classic case of chronic fatigue.

It was around this time that I had my first whiff of Wild Orange essential oil, and I thought I could simply replace my daily sugar and caffeine with a bottle of citrus—my new "energy bomb." What I soon learned was that essential oils can bridge the gap, but I needed an entire lifestyle makeover to reclaim the natural energy I needed.

The Why *Behind a Lack of Energy, and the Torture of Fatigue*

"I just need more energy!" is a phrase I hear from almost all my patients, and it's one of the biggest issues that women face today as they try to be everything for everyone. Unfortunately, there is no easy fix for this problem because, once you've hit the wall of fatigue and energy failure, your underlying issues need immediate attention. But there is hope and there are solutions!

The long-term goal is to have sustained energy over time so you can tackle whatever life throws at you. No one recipe or chapter in this book will solve all your problems—you have to be willing to invest in yourself to reclaim that energy, and the 14-Day Rescue Plan in Part III, with its comprehensive program of daily essential-oil use, good nutrition, supplementation, exercise, and self care, will be the beginning to your rebuilding process.

Your Hormones for Energy

Hormones work synergistically in your body, and when they are not in balance, your energy level will suffer. The best solution is *prevention*. Nurturing your body and staving off stress will work wonders to give you the energy you need.

Cortisol and Epinephrine

In the short term, epinephrine (aka-adrenaline) jumps the body into action to protect from potential stressors, releasing energy in the fight-or-flight response. Your body also triggers the adrenals to produce norepinephrine, making the body momentarily stronger, more alert, and full of energy.

As discussed in the previous chapter, chronic stress and excess cortisol causes a domino effect, wreaking havoc with the HPA axis and leading to adrenal fatigue and its attendant symptoms. In addition to the suggestions in Chapter 5, there are specific forms of exercise that have been proven to lower cortisol levels when done properly, as you'll see in Chapter 15. Conversely, *too much* exercise can cause your cortisol levels to rise; see more in the Self-Care Rituals on page 112.

Melatonin

The levels of the sleep hormone melatonin are triggered by darkness; they should rise in the evening hours and peak in the early morning hours, enabling you to get a restful night's sleep. As you will discover in Chapter 7, there are easy steps you can take to improve your sleep. Without enough uninterrupted sleep, as you are doubtless aware, you won't have optimal energy.

T4, T3, and TSH

These thyroid hormones manage the body's metabolism in order to convert glucose and fat into usable energy. Every cell of your body relies on this balance in order to properly function, so any stress placed on the thyroid will cause energy issues and fatigue. Hypothyroidism occurs when your body doesn't produce enough thyroid hormones, leaving you with decreased energy levels and pronounced fatigue. Depression, mood swings, sleep issues, and fatigue are all symptoms of hypothyroidism, as well as menopause—which is why they're often dismissed as solely menopausal and treated incorrectly, compounding the problem.

Since chronic stress affects the HPA axis, treating your body well will support your thyroid. In addition, a proper diet rich in selenium and iodine, as well as healthy fats like omega-3s, will provide nutritional support for your thyroid. Regulating blood sugar levels will help keep insulin resistance at bay; any blood sugar irregularities weaken thyroid function.

Estrogen and Progesterone

Balanced levels of estrogen and progesterone allow your reproductive system to properly function. Estradiol (E2) greatly impacts energy levels, as well as other functions such as sleep, libido, and growth. It also influences the production of serotonin levels.

As you will see in Chapters 9 and 14, a variety of endocrine disruptors (particularly toxins and xenoestrogens) can influence estrogen and progesterone levels, which in turn affects other hormones like serotonin. Chronic stress also lowers estradiol in the process. Symptoms include fatigue, headaches, insomnia, anxiety, low libido, and hot flashes.

Testosterone

Testosterone helps a woman's body stay balanced and contributes to a healthy libido, muscle strength, bone health, and a strong metabolism. Low levels of testosterone lead to a decreased libido and zapped energy. With those results, it's no wonder that depression is also a common symptom of low testosterone. High levels can cause acne, excess facial hair, and more serious conditions such as polycystic ovarian syndrome (PCOS).

Leptin and Ghrelin

Of these two important hormones for the regulation of satiety, ghrelin tells us how much to eat and leptin tells us when to stop. Leptin can also signal the use of adipose tissue (fat stores) for energy production, as it regulates appetite and balances energy in the body. Ghrelin aids in our energy metabolism on a long-term basis as well.

When we consume too much sugar, leptin production can stall, causing an amped-up production of ghrelin to make us think we're perpetually hungry. In addition, with low levels of leptin, the body goes into starvation mode, thinking that food must be consumed whenever it becomes available and causing a propensity for binge eating. Compound that with added stress, the binge eating and sugar spikes become a bad pattern that keeps the body moving. Cutting back on sugar and keeping your diet full of plant-based, whole-food selections can help regulate your hormones and keep energy levels balanced.

When Fatigue Becomes Chronic

Chronic fatigue syndrome (CFS) plagues many people with extreme fatigue yet who seemingly have no underlying medical condition or explanation. Rest rarely helps, although CFS does become exacerbated with physical or mental exertion. There is no one way to test for CFS, but it is often diagnosed after a laundry list of other issues have been eliminated. Since the cause is unknown, the best we can do is treat the symptoms.

Discussing your situation with a trusted health-care provider can assist you in developing a game plan for eliminating potentially life-threatening disorders and other illnesses, infections, immune system sensitivities, hormonal imbalances, or psychological issues. Be sure to discuss any concerns that you may have and advocate for yourself until you feel comfortable with whatever suggestions the doctor may have for you.

In my practice, I have found that building a healthy foundation of good diet, exercise, and adequate sleep, while reducing stress and supporting the body with essential oils, can greatly influence the effects of CFS. Resetting your body with the 14-Day Rescue Plan can help get it on the right track again, once your health-care provider has given you the go-ahead to try it.

Emotional Triggers

I'll admit, there were multiple occasions when I found myself easily triggered under stressful situations. During the height of my hormonal imbalance, I would overreact to the smallest things. These moments profoundly affected my overall mood and energy levels.

Over time, I learned to recognize my emotional triggers and I made positive strides to address them. I knew that when I felt overwhelmed and exhausted, it was time for me to step back from a triggering emotional situation, grab an essential oil (like Clary Sage), and take a couple deep breaths.

Stress and fatigue can easily become your new normal as your body adjusts to chronically high levels of cortisol and all of the symptoms that it causes. The longer you go on ignoring what your body is telling you, the easier it is to feel emotionally triggered.

In those moments, allow yourself grace. You are the CEO of your health and you have beautiful, effective tools to support you. It's time to rise above and revisit what you consider normal to support and sustain a happy mind and body!

How to Support Energy/ Fight Fatigue with Essential Oils

Essential oils with ketones and monoterpenes, such as limonene and beta-pinene, are incredible for lifting your mood and giving you energy boosts throughout the day—so you will never find me without at least one energy-boosting blend in my purse!

Preferred Essential Oils

CITRUS ESSENTIAL OILS

BERGAMOT (*Citrus bergamia*)

- Calms and uplifts the mind and body while alleviating fatigue, tension, and anxiety
- Perfect for massage blends and diffusing, as well as calm when added to black herbal tea

LEMON (*Citrus limon*)

- Promotes a positive mood while invigorating the mind and body
- Perfect addition to smoothies and water for internal support, detox, and digestion

LIME (*Citrus aurantifolia*)

- Stimulates the mind and body while uplifting mood and refreshing the senses
- Promotes emotional health and well-being
- Perfect addition to smoothies and recipes for internal support and detox

WILD ORANGE (*Citrus sinensis*)

- Energizing aroma that uplifts the mind and body while purifying the air
- Perfect addition to smoothies for internal support and detox

Aromatic Use

- Diffuse 2 drops with Peppermint and Frankincense, or other complementary essential oils. Use the recipes that follow as a guide.
- Breathe directly from the bottle.

Topical Use

- Add to massage blends or rollerball blends for an extra mood-lifting boost. (Remember that citrus oils are phototoxic, so avoid direct sunlight for at least 12 hours with most citrus oils but up to 72 hours with Bergamot.)

PEPPERMINT (*Mentha piperita*)

- Promotes energetic feelings by enlivening the senses
- Encourages healthy respiratory function to enhance your exercise routines
- Cools and invigorates skin helping to improve focus and alertness

Aromatic Use

- Diffuse 3–4 drops.
- Diffuse with Wild Orange for an amazing energy boost.

Topical Use

- Add 1 drop each of Peppermint, Wild Orange, and Frankincense to your palms, rub together, and inhale deeply.
- Dilute 1 part oil to 3 parts carrier oil, and massage onto neck and shoulders.
- Dilute 1 part oil to 3 parts carrier oil, and massage into fatigued and tense areas of the body.

ROSEMARY (*Rosmarinus officinalis*)

- Energizes and renews the mind and body while honing focus and memory
- Reduces nervous tension and aids in reducing symptoms of fatigue

Aromatic Use

- Diffuse 3–4 drops to create a relaxing environment.
- Apply 1 drop to palms, rub together, cup over nose, and deeply inhale.

Topical Use

- Dilute 1 part oil to 3 parts carrier oil, and massage into tense or stressed muscles.

EUCALYPTUS (*Eucalyptus radiata*)

- Clears and focuses the mind while opening the respiratory system
- Alleviates nervous tension and anxiousness

- Purifies the skin while invigorating the mind and body and enhancing vitality

Aromatic Use

- Diffuse 3–4 drops to open respiratory pathways. Especially effective during yoga or other anabolic exercise, or before catabolic exercise.
- Add 2 drops to a cotton ball or directly on floor during a steamy shower.
- Inhale directly from the bottle or add 1 drop in your palms, rub together, cup over nose, and inhale deeply. Rub remaining oil into your neck and shoulders for sustained benefits.

Topical Use

- Dilute 1 part oil into 3 parts of your favorite massage moisturizer.
- Add 1 drop to your favorite body wash.

FRANKINCENSE (*Boswellia carterii, B. frereana,* and *B. sacra*)

- Enhances a sense of peace and vitality while relaxing the mind and body
- Supports immune health and cellular function

Aromatic Use

- Diffuse 3–4 drops. Especially effective during yoga and other anabolic exercise.
- Add 1 drop Frankincense and 1 drop Wild Orange to palms, rub together, cup over nose, and inhale deeply. Add Peppermint for an even bigger energy boost.

Topical Use

- Dilute 1–2 drops with your favorite carrier oil and massage into the hands and body.
- Apply 1–2 drops with your favorite carrier oil to your soles at night.

BASIL (*Ocimum basilicum*)

- Enhances mental focus and alertness while rejuvenating the mind and body
- Alleviates nervous tension and anxiety in the mind and body

Aromatic Use

- Diffuse 3–4 drops.
- Inhale directly from the bottle.

Topical Use

- Apply 1 drop to fingertips and massage into temples.
- Dilute 1–2 drops with your favorite carrier oil and massage into tense muscles. Add 1 drop of Wintergreen for a cooling and relaxing sensation.

Angela's Story

Angela was a forty-nine-year-old college administrator and single mother of three children in high school. With all her children participating in high school activities, she felt drained after the end of each day, especially as weekends were filled with even more activities. Angela came to me needing a massive reset; she was overwhelmed and felt like she didn't recognize the woman in the mirror. Her diet had suffered and she had no energy by noon, and was surviving on chocolate and sugar to get through the day.

Angela presented with low cortisol levels in the morning and high cortisol levels in the evening, stress, poor diet, and overall burnout. **My recommendations were as follows:**

- For afternoon slumps, incorporate the Instant Energy Boost Ritual (page 112), or diffuse energizing essential oils such as the Energy Booster Diffuser Blend (page 105) or Fatigue Fighter Diffuser Blend (page 105).

- Crave-Control Rollerball Blend (page 147) in the afternoon to reduce chocolate cravings and boost energy.
- A 30-minute self-care morning ritual consisting of inhaling the Morning Boost Inhaler Blend (page 106), journaling, 5-minute meditation, green smoothie, and stretching, or yoga.
- Thirty-minute short-burst exercises to ramp up her metabolism and burn fat three times a week.
- Eliminating chocolate power bars and candy bars as snacks throughout the day, and substituting a green smoothie and green tea for breakfast and lunch.
- Following the 14-Day Rescue Meal Plan to reset eating habits and support healthy hormone changes.
- Supplements: a multivitamin, 300 mg of magnesium glycinate, 500 mg of ashwagandha, and 2000 mg of omega-3 fatty acids to lower stress levels and increase lean body mass.

Within a month, Angela experienced more energy, especially in the middle of the day and on weekends, and was enjoying that thirty minutes of her morning as belonging to just her. She lost eight pounds on the 14-Day Rescue Meal Plan, and she continued to cook many of the recipes from the plan; her kids even enjoyed them, which was a big win for her. Her chocolate cravings significantly decreased, and she didn't feel as dependent on sugar to get through her day. "The morning ritual was a game changer for me—I am so grateful to have a moment to focus on my health," she told me. "The essential oils have made all the difference with my cravings and energy levels. I feel confident that I can continue these routines and continue to see improvements in my health."

Essential Oil Blends

Aromatic Diffuser Blends

Energy Booster Diffuser Blend

2 drops Wild Orange essential oil
2 drops Douglas Fir essential oil
2 drops Peppermint essential oil

Fatigue Fighter Diffuser Blend

3 drops Eucalyptus essential oil
2 drops Rosemary essential oil
2 drops Lemongrass essential oil

Focus over Fatigue Diffuser Blend

1 drop Rosemary essential oil
3 drops Peppermint essential oil
3 drops Tangerine essential oil

Encourage and Uplift Diffuser Blend

2 drops Grapefruit (or any citrus oil) essential oil
2 drops Frankincense essential oil
1 drop Sandalwood essential oil

Invigorate and Vitalize Diffuser Blend

3 drops Tangerine essential oil
1 drop Basil essential oil
2 drops Spearmint essential oil

Aromatic Personal Inhaler Blends

Exercise Boost Inhaler Blend

4 drops Peppermint essential oil
4 drops Eucalyptus essential oil

2 drops Rosemary essential oil

2 drops Lemon essential oil

Morning Boost Inhaler Blend

5 drops Peppermint essential oil

3 drops Rosemary essential oil

5 drops Grapefruit essential oil

Motivate and Move Inhaler Blend

4 drops Wild Orange essential oil

4 drops Frankincense essential oil

4 drops Lemon essential oil

3 drops Spearmint essential oil

Aromatic Room Spray

Energizing Room Spray

15 drops Frankincense essential oil

15 drops Grapefruit, Lemon, or Wild Orange essential oil (or 5 drops each)

30 drops Douglas Fir essential oil

Distilled water

Add essential oils to a 2-ounce glass spray bottle and fill the rest with water. Cover and shake gently to combine. Spritz around your home.

Topical Rollerball Blends

Energy Booster Rollerball Blend

10 drops Peppermint essential oil

15 drops Wild Orange essential oil

Carrier oil of choice

Add the essential oils to a 10 mL glass rollerball bottle and fill the rest of the way with a carrier oil. Replace the rollerball top and cap, and shake gently to blend. To use, apply to pulse points, including behind the ears.

Get It Done Rollerball Blend

5 drops Rosemary essential oil
8 drops Peppermint essential oil
8 drops Wild Orange essential oil
6 drops Frankincense essential oil
Carrier oil of choice

Add the essential oils to a 10 mL glass rollerball bottle and fill the rest of the way with a carrier oil. Replace the rollerball top and cap, and shake gently to blend. To use, apply to pulse points, especially behind the ears and on the wrist, inhaling deeply when necessary to boost and focus.

Pre-Workout Rollerball Blend

8 drops Peppermint essential oil
8 drops Eucalyptus essential oil
4 drops Rosemary essential oil
4 drops Lavender essential oil
2 drops Wild Orange essential oil
Carrier oil of choice

Add the essential oils to a 10 mL glass rollerball bottle and fill the rest of the way with a carrier oil. Replace rollerball top and cap, and shake gently to blend. To use, roll behind the ears, and on pulse points.

Focus and Uplift Massage Rollerball Blend

5 drops Basil essential oil
10 drops Cypress essential oil
5 drops Grapefruit essential oil
5 drops Peppermint essential oil
Carrier oil of choice

Add the essential oils to a 10 mL glass rollerball bottle and fill the rest with a carrier oil. Replace the rollerball top and cap, then shake gently to combine. To use, roll on neck and shoulders and massage using smooth yet firm strokes.

Shower and Bath Blends

Invigorating Morning Bliss Shower Spray

10 drops Peppermint essential oil
5 drops Cedarwood essential oil
5 drops Wild Orange essential oil
3 tablespoons distilled water

Add the essential oils to a 2-ounce glass spray bottle and add the water. Replace the cap and shake to combine. Spritz 5–7 times in the shower. Breathe deeply.

Basic Shower and Bath Bomb

1 cup citric acid
1 cup baking soda
½ cup cornstarch or arrowroot powder
12–15 drops favorite essential oils, or one of the blends that follow
¼ to ⅓ cup water
Silicone mold of your choice, or mini cupcake pan (typically used for baking)

In a glass bowl, combine the citric acid, baking soda, and cornstarch or arrowroot powder, followed by the essential oils. Next, add the water a bit at a time, stirring—just enough water to make a soft dough. If the mixture is too wet, try adding a little more baking soda and cornstarch until consistency is correct. Gently press the mixture into the molds and let sit for at least 24 hours, testing first to see if the bombs are dry. Remove from the molds and store in an airtight container. To use, drop into the tub or shower and allow to dissolve.

Relax and Rejuvenate Bath Soak

3 drops Rosemary essential oil
3 drops Frankincense essential oil
3 drops Lavender essential oil
¼ cup Epsom salts
Warm water bath

Add the essential oils to the Epsom salts and swirl into a warm bath to dissolve.

Bath Bomb Blends

Breathe Easy Bath Blend

7 drops Eucalyptus essential oil
5 drops Lavender essential oil
3 drops Peppermint essential oil

Sunny Citrus Bath Blend

7 drops Bergamot essential oil
5 drops Wild Orange essential oil
3 drops Grapefruit essential oil

Internal Uses

Dehydration is often a culprit for energy drain. For momentary fatigue, first drink 8 to 16 ounces of water with an essential oil boost if you want extra flavor and energy. I recommend carrying water with you all day in a glass bottle or stainless steel jug as a continual reminder. I always try to drink at least 8 ounces of water with each meal, as well as during my mid-morning and mid-afternoon snack breaks. Aim for 8 to 10 glasses of water per day to stay properly hydrated.

Lemon-Strawberry Detox Water

1 cup hulled and sliced strawberries

1 lemon, sliced into wheels, pits removed

2 drops Lemon essential oil

Ice cubes

1½ quarts filtered water

Add the fruit and Lemon essential oil to a 2-quart glass pitcher. Add the desired amount of ice to the pitcher, then fill with the water. Refrigerate and allow to steep for at least 30 minutes, preferably for 2 to 3 hours, before enjoying.

Energy-Boosting Berry Infusion

2 cups fresh or frozen berries of choice (blueberries, blackberries, cherries, raspberries, etc.)

2 drops Lemon essential oil

Ice cubes

1½ quarts filtered water

Add the berries and essential oil to a 2-quart glass pitcher. Add the desired amount of ice to the pitcher, then fill with the water. Refrigerate and allow to steep for at least 30 minutes before enjoying.

Supplements to Support Energy and Reduce Fatigue

Proper supplementation can help support energy levels. Supplements are especially beneficial for those of us who are nutrient-deficient, either from not eating enough of the right foods or from eating foods with a lower nutritional composition. Be sure to discuss supplementation with your trusted health-care provider to ensure you are making the proper choices.

I recommend a daily supplement pack for heart, brain, and cellular support along with an energy supplement that assists with healthy mitochondrial function. My preference is a whole-food vitamin and mineral supplement, an omega-3 fatty acid, and a cellular and polyphenol antioxidant blend. This trio will also support healthy digestion and a healthy immune system, as well as an improved energy level. In addition, you may need the following:

Magnesium glycinate. A crucial component in our bodies, though most people are deficient in this vital mineral. In addition to supporting cellular energy levels, it supports the HPA axis by regulating healthy cortisol levels and protecting your body from toxins and free radicals. This helps to up your libido and promote fertility for a healthy reproductive system unencumbered by chronic stress levels. The Recommended Dietary Allowance (RDA) for magnesium is around 320 milligrams per day.

Iron. Critical for supplying oxygen to your body, iron keeps your energy steady. A common deficiency, low iron can leave you fatigued, weak, irritable, and unable to focus—what's often called "tired blood." Natural whole-food sources of iron include grass-fed meats and liver, lentils, chickpeas, spinach, and nuts. Do not self-diagnose, as too much iron can cause other problems; ask for a blood test ahead of supplementation.

Ashwagandha and Rhodiola Rosea. These two herbs in combination have been proven to help boost energy while strongly supporting adrenal function. As adaptogenic herbs, they can help fight stressors naturally while their rejuvenating properties can revitalize body and mind, renewing sustainable energy and combating fatigue. In addition, they offer immune support, fat-burning power, hormonal balance, and overall body balance.

Vitamin B$_{12}$. This vitamin that is essential for natural energy also helps with immune function, blood formation, DNA synthesis, and digestion. Deficiencies leave you feeling drained and easily fatigued, contributing to symptoms like muscle weakness, lack of focus and concentration, mood issues, and lack of motivation. As these symptoms can take years to manifest, supplementation now is a good idea.

Vitamin D. As with iron, we are often deficient in vitamin D, which can be obtained by getting at least 15 to 20 minutes of direct sunlight per day. You can also supplement your diet with fish such as salmon and mackerel, cod liver oil, egg yolks, and beef liver; since this list may be undesirable for some, supplements in the form of D3 should be considered. Vitamin D increases natural levels of dopamine and serotonin, essential for keeping mood balanced and favorable, and aids in many other functions, so make sure you're getting enough. (If your levels are normal, you need at least 400–800 IU per day.)

Self-Care Rituals for Supporting Energy and Reducing Fatigue

Instant Energy Boost Ritual

I have witnessed firsthand the power of one of the simplest blends I recommend: the Energy Booster Diffuser Blend (page 105). One deep breath immediately lifts your emotions, focuses your senses, and boosts your energy. One roll behind your ears allows for immediate absorption, facilitating sustained energy and vitality throughout the day. Consistent use of the blend trains your body to associate the scent with an immediate boost, so that you are never without an energy solution when you need one. Peppermint and Wild Orange essential oils will always be my favorite go-to's for a personal energy boost, but don't be afraid to experiment with the oils recommended in this chapter to find your own favorite blend.

Balanced Exercise Ritual

Cardiovascular exercise and strength training are the backbone of any fitness program, but as we age and our hormones shift, our bodies respond differently to the exercises. Shorter bursts of moderate-intensity exercise performed even twice a week, along with strength-training exercises, provide a greater post-exercise metabolic boost compared to longer, more frequent bouts of exercise at lower intensity. While all forms of exercise offer stress-reduction benefits, balancing your cardiovascular exercise with optimal amounts of strength training provides the benefits of cholesterol reduction, better blood sugar control, more effective body-fat reduction, and cardiovascular benefits.

Morning Smoothie Ritual

You already know how much I love my green smoothies (see pages 322 and 323)!

Coming Home Ritual

Your body needs some time to adjust and unwind after work. I recommend slipping into either comfortable clothes or a special pair of slippers. Turn on a welcome-home playlist, or find something that you enjoy, like cooking, reading, or taking that evening bath. This will validate the transition from work time to self-care time.

Fuel-Your-Body Ritual

Fueling your body the right way, with the best food options—a plant-based, whole-food diet with grass-fed animal protein—helps you to maintain natural energy levels. You need to view eating as a primary way to care for yourself. Eating every four to six hours will help balance your metabolism and maintain muscle mass, but only eat when you are hungry. Cutting out pseudo-energy items like caffeine, energy drinks, and especially sugar will have a huge impact on your energy levels. A food journal will help you track your eating patterns and triggers, so get writing!

CHAPTER 7

Sleep Issues

When was the last time you got at least seven hours of restful, uninterrupted, quality sleep? I'll admit, I'm guilty of trying to make my body run on less sleep than it needs. Between my busy schedule, intense amounts of travel between time zones, and the chaos of my daily life, I can very easily fall victim to the "wired and tired" craze that happens when I allow my hormones to become imbalanced from chronic stress and lack of restful sleep.

I know that you can get what you think is eight hours of good sleep, yet still wake up utterly exhausted because you've let your hormones become so imbalanced that your body can't recharge at night. My patients often have the same struggles as I do, depending on their stage in life and what they subject their bodies to in the course of the day. Many of them finally admit, "I'm so tired all the time, why is it so hard for me to fall asleep?"

What are the solutions we often choose? Caffeine. Carbs. Sleeping aids. Wine. All the things that actually don't help us achieve quality sleep at all.

Sleep is critical to our overall well-being, and the consequences of sleep deprivation can be life-threatening—and not just if you've nearly fallen asleep at the wheel. Our reflexes and concentration will be blunted, judgment impaired, temper frayed, mood depressed, energy zapped, and hormones unable to bounce back. Over time, the stress of it can completely do us in. Thanks to hormonal fluctuations during a menstrual cycle, and then the changes associated with decreasing hormone levels in perimenopause and menopause, our circadian rhythms can't compete. Add the outside influences such as busy schedules, computer screens at night, jet lag, even daylight savings, and we become chronically sleep-deprived.

The Why Behind Sleep Issues

Sleep health doesn't top the list of our health concerns, though our body's ability to revive and restore, as well as regulate hormonal levels and other functions, should put it at the top. In fact, many of us have no idea what a good night's sleep truly feels like because we have neglected our sleep health for so long.

Does everyone need the same amount of sleep? No, but everyone needs a certain amount of sustained *quality* sleep complete with deep REM (rapid eye movement) cycles. According to the National Sleep Foundation, the average adult needs seven to nine hours of sleep. How much you actually need depends on several factors, such as how you feel when you wake up; how long it takes you to fall asleep; the amount of stress, caffeine, or other factors that influence your body on a daily basis; and any chronic health issues that may be affecting you—at bare minimum.

A great way to test yourself: Practice a nighttime ritual to wind your body down, including no electronics, lowering the temperature in your bedroom, shutting off all extraneous lights, decreasing your caffeine and food intake prior to bedtime, and allowing your body to relax. Then shut off the alarm. Take note of the time you lie down in bed, practice deep-breathing techniques for calming down, and then see how long you sleep before you wake up. If you're already experiencing sleep issues, this may feel like an impossible task, but if you can complete this test, you will see where you fall along the seven-to-nine-hour spectrum.

Most important, if you are sleeping outside this normal range— more or less—you either have issues you are ignoring or you aren't allowing your body to get the sleep it needs. Sleep allows our hormones to regulate a variety of functions, and it affects our ability to regulate emotions, mood, and maintain proper energy levels, as well as influencing our appetite and ability to burn fat and balance blood sugar levels. Without enough sleep, our bodies don't have enough time to complete the cycles needed for optimal health.

Your Hormones for Sleep

Melatonin

Known as the "sleep hormone," melatonin is produced by the pineal gland in the brain, and its function is to regulate your sleep/wake cycle. The amount of melatonin your body makes is predicated on how much light you're exposed to during the day; normally, levels increase around two hours before your normal bedtime. Surprisingly, according to a study done at the University of Maryland Medical Center, melatonin affects a woman's menstrual cycle, including its regularity and onset of menstruation, as well as the start of menopause, by aiding in the timing and release of female reproductive hormones.

A structured bedtime routine helps keep melatonin levels on an even, predictable schedule, but this is often hampered by the blue light emitted by our electronic devices—it tricks the brain into thinking it's not nighttime and so the melatonin levels don't increase as they should. Shutting off your electronics for at least an hour before bedtime will greatly aid your ability to fall asleep.

Many people also self-medicate with melatonin supplements. I've found that they seem to either work very well or not at all.

Some users have reported side effects, such as vivid and disturbing dreams, or even more disrupted sleep. If so, discontinue their use. As always, consult a medical professional before taking any over-the-counter hormone, especially melatonin, as it is contraindicated with certain medications, such as birth control pills.

Estrogen

Estrogen levels naturally fluctuate during a menstrual cycle, which is why many women have sleep issues on the day before their period arrives, when levels are the lowest. As estrogen levels decrease during perimenopause and menopause, this can compound sleep issues. One of the reasons for this is estrogen's influence on how well the tissues and bones can absorb magnesium, which is an important component for sleep regulation, as it aids in melatonin processing. Less estrogen means less efficient magnesium metabolism.

Cortisol

Normally, cortisol levels should decrease in the evening just as melatonin is increasing, remain low throughout the night, and then gradually begin to increase in order to wake you up in the morning. It should come as no surprise that cortisol affects your ability to enter into restful and sustained sleep. After all, if danger threatens to attack at any given moment, how could your body relax enough to go into a deep sleep? Chronic stress hijacking your HPA axis affects your ability to fall asleep and sink into that deep, restful REM sleep you need to recharge.

Interestingly, studies have shown that insomniacs have increased levels of ACTH (adrenocorticotropic hormone) in their bloodstream, indicating that chronic stress directly correlates to severe inability to both fall asleep and maintain a restful sleep pattern throughout the night.

Growth Hormone

Growth hormone produced in the pituitary gland is released during sleep so the body can continue to grow and develop, and to aid in the repair of damaged tissues. Though more pertinent during childhood and adolescence, growth hormone can still be a factor if you've had disrupted sleep since those years. Adolescents are chronically sleep-deprived, which can potentially cause detrimental effects on their growth and development. Increased stress on the HPA axis can also potentially threaten growth hormone's normal release.

Ghrelin, Leptin, and Insulin

The "hunger hormones" need you to sleep in order to balance your natural appetite. Ghrelin stimulates hunger patterns, and sleep regulates these levels, so sleeping poorly will actually make you feel hungrier. Likewise, leptin inhibits hunger in order to regulate body weight; when its levels are regulated at night during sleep, we don't get hungry while we rest. If you aren't getting proper amounts of quality sleep, it's easier to gain weight, as your hunger levels won't be properly balanced.

In addition, the body should follow a natural pattern of rising and falling cortisol and insulin levels so that we wake up hungry and properly nourish our body. Insulin aids in controlling glucose levels, as well as regulating carbohydrate and fat metabolism. Allowing these hormones to do their job during sleep helps their normal function during the day.

Prolactin

Produced in the pituitary gland, prolactin is a hormone that influences over 300 bodily functions, most notably immune system function. Higher levels are released during sleep, so if you're not getting enough sleep, this can mean a weakened immune system.

The importance of sleep can't be overstated. Creating your own

Sometimes You've Just Got to Go in the Middle of the Night

As you'll see in Chapter 9 (page 151), one of the common symptoms of perimenopause and menopause is an overactive bladder. You might find yourself waking up out of a deep sleep to go to the bathroom as you get older, whether you truly have to pee or not. Many women suffer in silence because they're too embarrassed to bring this up with their medical professionals.

The nighttime need to pee is due to aldosterone, which causes water retention. Produced in the adrenal cortex, aldosterone should remain high during sleep to prevent nighttime urination, but fluctuating progesterone levels can cause a decrease in its levels, leading to a lessened ability to retain water.

Once your hormones are better regulated, you should experience some improvement. Don't cut down on your water intake, as hydration plays a role in keeping your entire body balanced. This blend is designed to give support to your kidneys and urinary tract, and it should give you some relief from nighttime urgency.

Bladder Boost Rollerball Blend

15 drops Cypress essential oil
15 drops Juniper Berry essential oil
Carrier oil of choice

Add the essential oils to a 10 mL glass rollerball bottle and fill the rest with your choice of carrier oil. Replace the rollerball top and shake gently to blend. To use, roll over the abdomen before bedtime to prevent urinary incontinence.

nighttime routine complete with essential-oil-supported sleep rituals can help you to get to the bottom of the hormonal issues that may be plaguing your circadian rhythms. The potency of my favorite, time-tested essential oils for sleep support never ceases to astound me. Remember that experimentation is the only way to figure out the best combination and application techniques that work for you. Keeping your favorite oils and blends on your bedside table can help you to establish and maintain a sleep routine, as well as be ready for those middle-of-the-night wakefulness situations.

Emotional Triggers

Emotions often play a big role in our sleep routines, but more often that's because they trigger our stress levels. For me, mental chatter due to stress and never-ending to-do lists keeps me up too often. The next day, the lack of sleep feels like a heavy weight on my body.

The good news is that essential oils can transport you from emotional distress to a healthy sleep pattern and on to a healthier you. Merely inhaling the scent of an essential oil can instantly lift your emotions, ground your mind and body, and enable you to follow a sleep routine that trains your body to relax and prepares you for deep, restful, rejuvenating sleep.

How to Support Your Sleep with Essential Oils

Each of the essential oils in this list was selected for its ability to promote relaxation and sleep; their primary constituents are either relaxing or have a sedative-like effect.

Preferred Essential Oils

BERGAMOT (*Citrus bergamia*)

- Calming and soothing to the mind and body, especially when used in massage
- Alleviates feelings of stress and anxiousness
- Known as the "self-assurance" and "self-love" oil

Aromatic Use

- Diffuse at night with one of the calming oils.
- Use one of the aromatic room sprays to spritz onto bedclothes and pillows before bedtime.

Topical Use

- Dilute 1–2 drops with a carrier oil and use as a pre-bedtime massage by rubbing into bottoms of feet, legs, back, and any area tight from tension. Or try the Nighttime Foot Mask (page 129)!
- Add to natural body wash during a warm shower and massage into skin.

CEDARWOOD (*Juniperus virginiana*)

- Natural sedative due to its primary constituent, cedrol
- May naturally relax the autonomic nervous system to soothe the body
- Grounding and calming for the mind and body

Aromatic Use

- Diffuse 3–4 drops at the end of the day.
- Inhale straight from the bottle.

Topical Use

- Add a drop to your nighttime natural facial moisturizer.
- Dilute 1–2 drops with your favorite carrier oil and apply to your soles before bed.

CLARY SAGE (*Salvia sclarea*)

- Promotes relaxation of the body for a restful night's sleep
- Calms and soothes the mind and body
- Supportive during menstrual distress

Aromatic Use

- Apply 1–2 drops directly to bedclothes or pillow.
- Diffuse 3–4 drops before bedtime.

Topical Use

- Dilute 1–2 drops with your favorite carrier oil and massage into abdomen.
- Add 2–3 drops to a warm bath with ¼ cup Epsom salts dissolved in the water.
- Dilute 1–2 drops with your favorite carrier oil and massage into your soles before bedtime.

LAVENDER (*Lavandula angustifolia*)

- Used as a sedative, to reduce anxious feelings, and to ease stress
- May slow down central nervous system activity and assist in serotonin release, resulting in calm in body and mind to support sleep
- Decreases blood pressure and supports restful night's sleep

Aromatic Use

- Diffuse 2–3 drops before bedtime, and add one of the complementary oils listed here to amp up the calming effect.
- Apply 1–2 drops directly to bedclothes and pillows before bedtime.

Topical Use

- Add 2–3 drops of Lavender and ½ cup Epsom salts to a warm bath.
- Dilute 1–2 drops with your favorite carrier oil and massage directly into your soles and on your chest.

Internal Use

- Add 1 drop of Lavender to ⅔ cup melted dark chocolate and stir well. Drop by teaspoonfuls onto wax paper or a silicone mat, or pour into a silicone mold. Allow to harden and enjoy one disk as a part of your nighttime mindfulness ritual.

ROMAN CHAMOMILE (*Anthemis nobilis*)

- Decreases levels of ACTH caused by stress to help induce relaxation
- Calms the mind, body, and skin while soothing bodily systems
- Supports a healthy immune system and soothes overall bodily systems

Aromatic Use

- Diffuse 2–3 drops before bedtime. Add 2 drops of Cedarwood essential oil for an extra calming environment.
- Inhale directly.
- Apply 1 drop of your favorite carrier oil to palms and rub together, cup over mouth and nose, and inhale deeply during moments of extreme tension or emotion.

Topical Use

- Dilute 1–2 drops with your favorite carrier oil and massage into any areas with pain-causing inflammation.
- Dilute 1–2 drops with your favorite carrier oil and apply to your soles.
- Dilute 1–2 drops with your favorite carrier oil and apply over pulse points.

SANDALWOOD (HAWAIIAN) (*Santalum paniculatum*)

- Calms and balances emotions as well as the mind and body
- Alleviates feelings of tension and pent-up emotions
- Promotes relaxation of the mind and body for a restful night's sleep

Aromatic Use

- Diffuse 3–4 drops during meditation at the end of the day.
- Diffuse 3–4 drops at bedtime.
- Apply 1 drop of your favorite carrier oil to palms, rub together, cup over mouth and nose, and inhale deeply before bedtime.

Topical Use

- Add 2–3 drops to ½ cup Epsom salts dissolved in a warm bath.
- Dilute 1–2 drops with your favorite carrier oil and massage into your neck and back.

VETIVER (*Vetiveria zizanioides*)

- Calms and grounds emotions, especially when used in massage
- Promotes a deep, restful night's sleep
- Supports a healthy immune system when taken internally

Aromatic Use

- Diffuse 3–4 drops before bedtime. Add 1–2 drops of Lavender to support sleep.
- Inhale directly from the bottle.

Topical Use

- Dilute 1–2 drops with your favorite carrier oil and massage into neck, shoulders, and soles before bedtime.
- Add 2–3 drops to ½ cup Epsom salts dissolved in a warm bath.

YLANG YLANG (*Cananga odorata*)

- Calming effect on mind and body while promoting positive moods
- Lessens stressful tension
- Promotes a healthy immune system with antioxidant support

Aromatic Use

- Diffuse 1–2 drops with Vetiver, Cedarwood, or Lavender before bedtime.

Topical Use

- Add 2–3 drops to ½ cup Epsom salts dissolved in a warm bath.

Pamela's Story

Pamela was forty-seven years old when she came to me, concerned with chronic exhaustion that she had been struggling with for over five years. Her biggest issue was falling asleep at night, despite trying supplements and sleeping pills. As an attorney, she often had to work late into the night, and the cases she managed kept her up due to stress and mental chatter.

Pamela was suffering from chronic stress, high cortisol levels, exhaustion, and brain fog. **My recommendations were as follows:**

- For afternoon slumps, a combination of Peppermint and Wild Orange essential oils for focus.
- For brain fog and concentration, the Motivation Rollerball Blend (page 222) and Rosemary essential oil, applied topically and aromatically.
- For sleep, the Mental Chatter Silencer Inhaler Blend (page 127) two hours before bed. She also used the Restful Sleep Room Spray (page 128) along with diluted Lavender and Clary Sage on her neck and feet before going to bed.
- The 30-minute Wind Down to Sleep Ritual (page 130) before bed to reduce stress and to relax her body before sleep.
- Yoga and Pilates three to four times a week for stress reduction.
- Substituting coffee with tea in the afternoon and evening.
- Recommended supplements: a multivitamin, 320 mg magnesium glycinate, 500 mg ashwagandha, and 2000 mg omega-3 fatty acids to lower stress

levels and support brain function. For sleep, 180–250 mg valerian and 42–60 mg hops.

It took less than a month for Pamela to gain more energy and, most important, she was getting at least seven hours of sleep each night. The modifications to her daily habits and sleep routine not only helped her recharge but also restored her relationship with her husband. She started focusing more on her health, and she felt the difference in her passion for life. "I am so grateful to have these simple rituals each day," she told me. "I never realized how essential oils and small lifestyle changes could have such a big impact on my life!"

Essential Oil Blends

Aromatic Diffuser Blends

Start your relaxing ritual at sundown by getting your diffusers going as soon as you come home from work. Running diffusers two to three hours before bedtime will help to calm your mind and give your body the signal that it's time to wind down.

Grounding Diffuser Blend

3 drops Roman Chamomile essential oil
2 drops Cedarwood essential oil
1 drop Lavender essential oil

Restful Relaxation Diffuser Blend

2 drops Ylang Ylang essential oil
2 drops Bergamot essential oil
1 drop Roman Chamomile essential oil

Nighty-Night Diffuser Blend

2 drops Clary Sage essential oil
2 drops Cedarwood essential oil
2 drops Yarrow essential oil

Deep Relaxation Diffuser Blend

3 drops Lavender essential oil
1 drop Vetiver essential oil
1 drop Roman Chamomile essential oil

Aromatic Personal Inhaler Blends

Calm the Storm Inhaler Blend

4 drops Wild Orange essential oil
4 drops Cedarwood essential oil
4 drops Lavender essential oil
3 drops Clary Sage essential oil

Soothe Me to Sleep Inhaler Blend

4 drops Lavender essential oil
4 drops Vetiver essential oil
3 drops Bergamot essential oil
3 drops Marjoram essential oil

Mental Chatter Silencer Inhaler Blend

5 drops Lavender essential oil
5 drops Vetiver essential oil
5 drops Clary Sage essential oil

Peaceful Sleep Inhaler Blend

8 drops Lavender essential oil
4 drops Hawaiian Sandalwood essential oil
4 drops Bergamot essential oil
2 drops Ylang Ylang essential oil

Aromatic Room and Body Spray

Restful Sleep Room Spray

10 drops Lavender essential oil
10 drops Cedarwood essential oil
5 drops Vetiver essential oil
¼ cup distilled water or witch hazel

In a 2-ounce glass spray bottle, combine the essential oils followed by the water or witch hazel. Cover and shake gently. Shake and spritz on pillows, comforters, and in the air before bed.

Topical Rollerball Blends

Sweet Dreams Rollerball Blend

10 drops Lavender essential oil
6 drops Vetiver essential oil
4 drops Yarrow essential oil
4 drops Ylang Ylang essential oil
Carrier oil of choice

Add the essential oils to a 10 mL glass rollerball bottle. Fill to the top with the carrier oil. Replace the rollerball top and cap, and shake gently to blend. To use, apply to your soles and pulse points.

Quiet Your Mind for Sleep Rollerball Blend

10 drops Lavender essential oil
5 drops Vetiver essential oil
5 drops Frankincense essential oil
4 drops Ylang Ylang essential oil

Add the essential oils to a 10 mL glass rollerball bottle. Fill to the top with the carrier oil. Replace the rollerball top and cap, and shake gently to blend. To use, apply to back of neck and your soles before bed.

Tension Release Rollerball Blend

8 drops Lavender essential oil

6 drops Cedarwood essential oil

6 drops Roman Chamomile essential oil

4 drops Clary Sage essential oil

3 drops Wintergreen essential oil

Carrier oil of choice

Add the essential oils to a 10 mL glass rollerball bottle. Fill to the top with the carrier oil. Replace the rollerball top and cap, and shake gently to blend. To use, apply to back of neck, down chest, and to any other tense areas before bed.

Personal Care Blend

Nighttime Foot Mask

Though it may seem odd to "mask" your feet, the ingredients in this recipe will prep you for bed and soothe those sore tootsies! Greek yogurt contains powerful probiotics to supply proteins and lactic acid as it sloughs off dead skin cells, while the vitamins and minerals in celery both nourish cracked skin and detox the body. Raw organic honey is packed with antioxidants and enzymes to support your body, and its anti-inflammatory properties are an added bonus. The trio of essential oils will help your body to find a natural calm and de-stress before bed.

1 organic celery stalk

½ cup plain organic Greek yogurt

2 tablespoons raw organic honey

2 teaspoons organic cold-pressed coconut oil

4 drops Bergamot essential oil

2 drops Lavender essential oil

2 drops Roman Chamomile essential oil

Grate the celery and pat dry with a paper towel. Add the celery, the yogurt, honey, and coconut oil to a blender or food processor and blend until smooth. Gently stir in the essential oils. Apply the mask immediately to your feet with your fingers or a soft-bristled brush, massaging in to cover entire area. Relax for 15 to 20 minutes with meditation or prayer, and then rinse off in the tub.

Self-Care Rituals for Sleep

Wind Down to Sleep Ritual

Our sleep success depends on the patterns and rituals we establish early on in life and carry out as we mature. Known as sleep hygiene, the things that we do to prepare for and sustain our sleep are part of caring for and keeping our bodies in top condition. Active preparation for sleep allows your body and mind to wind down and prepare for the act, instead of collapsing into bed like so many of us do thanks to our nonstop active lives.

Just as if you were a baby fresh into this world, you create a nighttime ritual to nurture yourself to sleep. A soothing bath; calming your mind with a book, meditation, or prayer; sipping a cup of tea; and working your essential oils to your benefit can all be a part of your calming routine. The key is to do these rituals every night at the same time so that your body gets used to them. Here's how to prepare your environment for proper sleep hygiene:

Darkness. No nightlights, no window light, no TV screens, and no electronic devices, please! Keep your room as dark as possible so that your brain can trigger the production of melatonin and help whisk you to sleep. If you do have issues with darkness, try using orange or red lightbulbs before sleep to calm your mind and also in the sleep zone when you do wake up.

Put the Electronic Devices Away. The blue light emitted from electronic devices is the enemy of sleep. Cellphones, tablets, TVs, computer monitors, and anything else with a bright screen can wake up your brain, especially if you've made it a part of your crawl-into-bed-and-check-my-social-media-one-last-time routine!

Temperature. Lowering the temperature of your house at night helps slow your heart rate and relax your body, preparing it for sleep. A programmable thermostat is a fantastic option if you don't have one already. Find a comfortable low somewhere between 68 and 70 degrees Fahrenheit (19–21 degrees Celsius) that doesn't make you uncomfortable, or have your thermostat adjust after your normal bedtime so it is virtually unnoticeable.

No Stimulants. Cut out caffeine, chocolate, coffee, nicotine, and anything else that might affect your ability to unwind. Even something as seemingly harmless as an all-natural super-minty peppermint toothpaste or mouthwash right before bed can wake you right up!

No Alcohol. That evening drink may seem to be the perfect cure for dulling your senses and making you drowsy, but it can become a problem in the long term, especially if your body begins to rely on it. The quantity that you drink and its frequency can be huge red flags for normal sleep, as your liver needs to metabolize the alcohol and, when completed, may disrupt your REM sleep by causing you to wake up or toss and turn throughout the night.

Say No to Late-night Snacks. While a high-protein choice containing tryptophan, an amino acid that supports serotonin and melatonin production, several hours before bedtime may help sustain you through the night, late-night or midnight snacks can keep you from sleep while your body works to digest what you ate and drank. In addition, many people find that they gain weight if they have a habit of eating right before bedtime, because they tend to overeat. If you want to support serotonin and melatonin levels, try a tryptophan booster at dinner like turkey, almonds, walnuts, sunflower seeds, hummus, or pumpkin seeds—snacks that are high in protein and low in sugar to sustain your nighttime cravings.

Nighttime Self-Care Ritual

Follow these steps to create a new, much healthier ritual:

Herbal Tea Time. Heat up water for your favorite herbal tea, like Roman Chamomile tea (without any added sugar!).

Healthy Snack Presentation. If you always crave something sweet at night, try replacing it with something healthier. Thinly slice an apple and fan the pieces out on your favorite plate. Pay attention to presentation to make this ritual a special occasion—we eat with our eyes first, and you deserve a little something special in the evening! Next, sprinkle the apples with cinnamon or your favorite spice. (Saigon cinnamon is perfectly sweet and pairs well with apples.) You can also soak the apples in a bowl with water and a few drops of Cinnamon Bark or Cassia essential oil for a juicy, spicy alternative. Eat slowly and mindfully. Sometimes, I add a small handful of almonds to avoid an insulin spike before going to bed.

Detox Bath. Begin a ritual of purposefully allowing yourself to unwind in a warm bath supported by the power of high-quality essential oils. Meditate on your day, pray, practice mindfulness, or just BE YOURSELF. Let the water slowly soak your stress away and allow the troubles to swirl down the drain when you're finished relaxing. Be sure to drink a glass of water afterward to rehydrate. Use the Relax and De-stress Bath Blend (page 164) to enhance this ritual.

Deep Breathing. As mentioned in previous chapters, deep breathing signals that everything is okay as it allows you to naturally unwind. Don't forget to rest in the pauses and allow yourself to experience the calm. Adding essential oils to this ritual will greatly enhance its power.

The Goodnight HUG. Before you enter your bedroom or as you lie down and begin to relax, you might find meditation and/or prayer can be extremely helpful in creating that calm. I recommend a guided routine of lows and highs to release any pent-up emotions that may have arisen during the day. Adding an essential-oil routine or diffuser to this time can also help. Close your eyes and focus on:

- **H—Heal.** Focus on areas that need healing in your life and positively reflect on things you have learned from this struggle.
- **U—Unwind.** Clock through your day and release any stressful situations one by one. It's over and done with, so leave your

worry in today's time while uplifting yourself to face tomorrow head-on.

- **G—Gratitude.** End your meditation with praise and thankfulness for things in your life, no matter how small, no matter how seemingly insignificant.

Calming Nighttime Meditation/Prayer Rollerball Blend

Essential oils have traditionally been used to support healthy meditation and prayer for centuries. This particular blend is meant to provide calm and peace to promote a restful night's sleep.

6 drops Frankincense essential oil
4 drops Clary Sage essential oil
4 drops Sandalwood essential oil
4 drops Lavender essential oil
2 drops Wild Orange essential oil
Carrier oil of choice

Add the essential oils to a 10 mL glass rollerball bottle and top off with your carrier oil of choice. Replace the rollerball and top, and shake gently to combine. Roll on your pulse points before bed. (The blend can also be reduced to 1 drop each and put in an ultrasonic diffuser.)

CHAPTER 8

Weight Issues

While you may assume that your weight problems are an inescapably normal part of age-related hormonal changes, there is a deeper, often-overlooked issue at play. Forget everything you've heard about the advertised fad diets—everything from where your weight gain is distributed to the cravings that you can't seem to shake can be related to hormones.

When normally fluctuating hormones tip the scale into an imbalance, a domino effect occurs in the body. While one system may be the only one showing symptoms for a while, soon you find yourself feeling out of control as one system after another succumbs to the effects of imbalanced hormones. What most women encounter, however, is that their symptoms so often appear to be something else to doctors who either treat only the surface issues or don't take the time to investigate the root cause of the problem. This is why it is crucial to treat each woman as a unique person, with her own history, emotions, and hormonal chemistry at play.

The Why *Behind Hormonal Weight Issues and Cravings*

Before our hormonal levels begin to naturally decline, we are used to experiencing cravings that kick into high gear when we are stressed, anxious, or at different stages in our menstrual cycle. We crave sugar and carbohydrates that help to ease stress levels during these tense times. Sugar has been shown to diminish physiological responses normally produced in the brain and body during stressful situations—not exactly great news for those of us who enjoy eating our feelings! And as was discussed in Chapter 5, the problem comes when we are chronically exposed to stress and we let our bodies and minds be tortured by it.

We also need to realize that *what* we crave isn't as important as *why* we crave. We are prone to eat in different ways as our hormonal levels change, but the reason for this will lead us to solutions for how to reset our bodies. There are different hormonal players at hand in the weight game, and each holds an important role in keeping our bodies healthy and balanced.

Your Hormones for Weight Issues and Cravings

Estrogen and Progesterone

While many people refer to these two as the sex hormones, it's important to understand that there are actually estrogen receptors all over your body. Reproductive system aside, estrogen plays a large role in your cardiovascular, musculoskeletal, immune, and central nervous systems as well. In particular, the estrogen receptors located in the brain's hypothalamus serve as a master switch that controls three important areas: food intake, energy expenditure, and body-fat distribution. When those estrogen levels begin to decline as we approach menopause, they are no longer able to regulate those three areas like they used to.

If you're gaining weight around your midsection, you know exactly what I'm talking about. You're not alone! Most women do gain midsection weight at this stage of life because lower estrogen levels trigger the body to shift fat from the hips and thighs to the belly area. According to a study reported by the Mayo Clinic in 2013, this shift also revs up the fat cells to store *more* fat just when you don't need it.

Estrogen, particularly **estradiol**, can decrease the amount of food we feel like eating and make us feel more satisfied after a meal. The problem comes when the body's estrogen levels begin to naturally decline and we are still accustomed to eating a certain amount. The brain may be sending signals that we just aren't quite full enough and we aren't left feeling as satisfied as we used to after a meal.

Ghrelin is another hormone that affects our eating routines, telling us that we need to eat. As we feed our bodies, ghrelin production decreases and estradiol sends messages to the brain that we aren't hungry anymore. With less estrogen, however, these communications systems aren't as quick to fulfill our needs as they once were.

Progesterone levels also decrease as age increases, causing us to retain water and experience bloating. While bloat may seem like weight gain, it is another annoying issue thanks to hormonal imbalance. Progesterone also has a calming effect on the brain that helps us to sleep, so it makes sense that decreased levels of progesterone lead to restlessness and sleep deprivation. What do we do when we can't sleep and find ourselves bored? Bring on the chocolate!

Insulin

You may be shocked to see *insulin* as a major player, especially if you aren't diabetic. What many of us misunderstand is that insulin is a vital part of our body chemistry. Produced by the pancreas, insulin is released into the body when we eat any form of carbohydrate, which the body then converts into glucose. Insulin's job is to transport the glucose through our bloodstream to all of the cells that need it for energy.

But when we consume *too much* carbohydrate, causing us to have excess glucose in our bloodstream, the body converts it to glycogen, which is then stored in the liver or, in the case of gross excess, stored as *fat*. Owing to poor diet and lack of exercise in our modern world, insulin resistance now dominates our culture, causing a whole host of issues.

Insulin functions as a key that needs to fit into the cell's lock to allow the glucose fuel to enter. When the receptors don't recognize it, the cells resist, refusing the fuel that they need to function. The body responds by decreasing our metabolism and draining our energy levels to preserve itself.

This translates into *self-inflicted starvation mode*. When our cells can't get the fuel that they need, they rely on fat stores instead. The body literally will not allow us to lose weight in favor of saving itself. No amount of reduced calories or strictest fad diet will help you to lose this weight until you can get your cells to accept the insulin again.

But what insulin resistance *does* cause is increased sugar and carbohydrate cravings that can be very hard to control. The body knows that it needs that glucose to survive, but the insulin resistance is just not permitting it to get through. Thus, we continue with the starvation/fat storage cycle.

The Estrogen–Insulin Connection

When estrogen levels naturally decline due to age, most of us put on a bit of weight because we continue to eat normally. We don't feel the insulin resistance beginning to take hold because there aren't yet major symptoms that arise like red flags. But they're there, keeping our cells from fueling up. As a result, they put a death grip on every last calorie that we consume and on the fat cells that store the glycogen. Storing the fat = survival!

If we don't start decreasing the amount of calories we eat when our estrogen levels begin to decline, we *will* gain weight. The problem is the fat now getting stored in the midsection—it's also getting stored around the organs. It secretes hormones called *adipokines*, which can increase our insulin resistance and also increase the risk of inflammation. They circulate throughout the body, communicating with other organs. *Leptin* is one of these adipokines that should signal satiety to the brain, but too much leptin owing to an excess of stored fat leaves the body without the "fullness" messages it needs. The result is that we never feel full or satisfied when we eat.

In addition, an insulin-resistant pancreas cannot manage extra sugar and a scary fact unfolds: the chronic hyper-secretion of insulin leads directly to heart disease.

Adrenaline and Cortisol—the STRESS Connection

It's no mystery that excess stress is directly related to weight gain, but exactly how this happens and the detrimental effect that chronic stress plays in our expanding waistlines may be surprising. It all comes back to our adrenals, the same glands responsible, along with the ovaries, for producing estrogen and progesterone. As you know already, the adrenal glands play a huge role in stress regulation as well, with *adrenaline* sending us into the fight-or-flight response and then *cortisol* shutting down systems in favor of self-preservation.

Years of chronic stress may have become your new normal and you can't seem to escape from it. "Rushing Women's Syndrome" and environmental threats compound this response. Already dealing with imbalanced hormones and now wacky body chemistry allow your metabolism to suffer. And then menopause begins to take hold.

After years of a famine-like state owing to chronic stress, our bodies may have become accustomed to the whirlwind of food that we subject it to. If our bodies constantly think they are in a state of famine, anytime food appears, it triggers an "Eat It All" response because we may never have the chance to eat again. Enter cravings, binges, and uncontrollable weight gain.

As our bodies break down muscle to fuel themselves, there is less muscle mass available to return excess glucose to. It deposits as body fat around our middles to protect our vital organs. Dieting does nothing but send more signals to our bodies that food is even scarcer than we thought.

Emotional Triggers

Consistent abuse of our stress hormones leads to chronic fatigue, grinds down our immune system and metabolism, and leads to even riskier situations, like Type 2 diabetes and heart disease. It makes our bodies feel burnt out, tired, fatigued, and stiff; and it affects our mental state and moods, leaving us with depression and anxiety-like symptoms.

Cravings are our bodies' fun way of signaling neglect or hormonal imbalance, but we train ourselves to use them as a coping mechanism. Whatever personal needs we ignore may turn into cravings to fill the voids. I call this "feeding an unmet need." That need can be emotional, physical, and even chemical. The immediate little "something" might help in the moment, but the craving doesn't address the core issue—it's only the *reaction* to it. The cravings won't go away until you figure out and address what the true triggers are, as well as the root cause of your problem.

Society has also conditioned us to use unhealthy food as a reward and comfort mechanism. When we celebrate, when we achieve a goal, when we find a personal success, when sadness envelops us, when tragedy strikes, when stress consumes us, we eat.

To manage cravings, you need to be able to identify true physical hunger from emotional hunger, and figure out what is driving that unmet need. Did you skip a meal? Is it energy? Is it stress? Is it a ritual that you created with friends, or loved ones? Boredom? Frustration? Procrastination? Sadness? Tracking your food consumption will help you to discover these emotional triggers for eating.

How to Support Weight Loss and Control Cravings with Essential Oils

A famous research study in the *Journal of Neurological and Orthopaedic Medicine and Surgery* by Dr. Alan Hirsch highlighted the amazing power of Peppermint essential oil. Hirsch found that Peppermint was able to combat food cravings while still perking up the senses and allowing the mind to focus. This makes Peppermint a perfect choice to keep your cravings away while changing your focus from that sugar binge to the task at hand. And Peppermint isn't the only oil with the potential to support your body through hormonal imbalance.

Even more essential oils have been studied and found effective at supporting a healthy weight. They are one of the easiest ways to sustain your metabolism, recover from years of hormonal abuse, and curb those emotional cravings. For each oil described here, you will find the scientific name helpful in choosing the best oil to support your weight loss and control your cravings, as well as suggestions on aromatic, topical, and internal applications, where appropriate.

Preferred Essential Oils

CASSIA (*Cinnamomum cassia*)
- Helps to stabilize blood sugar levels
- Promotes feelings of fullness and satiety
- Supports healthy digestion and immune function

Aromatic Use
- Combine 1–2 drops in a diffuser with citrus oils or Ginger.

WARNING: Use caution with direct inhalation, as it can be an overly strong scent.

Topical Use
- Create a warming massage by applying diluted Cassia to tense areas or to areas of concern.

WARNING: Always dilute Cassia with 1–2 drops per teaspoon of carrier oil, as it is a warming oil and can cause irritation.

CINNAMON BARK (*Cinnamomum zeylanicum*)

- Naturally helps to boost heart health
- Suppresses appetite and minimizes bingeing
- Fights sugar cravings by regulating blood glucose levels
- Supports a healthy metabolism and immune system

Aromatic Use

- Diffuse 1–2 drops.

WARNING: Use caution with direct inhalation, as it can be an overly strong scent.

Topical Use

- Create a warming massage by applying diluted Cinnamon Bark directly to tense areas.

WARNING: Always dilute Cinnamon Bark with 1–2 drops per teaspoon of carrier oil, as it is a warming oil and can cause irritation.

Internal Use

- Dip a toothpick in the Cinnamon Bark bottle then swirl into 2 cups of hot water or tea, and drink slowly at night.

BERGAMOT (*Citrus bergamia*)

- Reduces feelings of anxiousness and stress to counteract emotional eating
- May reduce cortisol levels
- Contains high levels of polyphenols, which combat fat and excess sugar

Aromatic Use

- Add 3–4 drops to a diffuser.
- Add a drop to your shower floor.

Topical Use

- Apply diluted to your soles at night.

WARNING: Bergamot is extremely phototoxic; avoid sun exposure for at least 72 hours after application.

Internal
- Dip a toothpick in the Bergamot oil bottle, then swirl into 1 cup of regular black tea to transform it into Earl Grey tea.

DILL (*Anethum graveolens*)
- Fights sugar cravings
- Supports healthy digestion and gastrointestinal health

Aromatic Use
- Diffuse 3 drops with 2 drops each Bergamot and Lemon.

Topical Use
- Apply, diluted, directly to your soles and massage in.
- To combat sugar cravings, dilute with a carrier oil and apply with a rollerball to wrists.

FENNEL (*Foeniculum vulgare*)
- Balances blood sugar levels
- Combats sugar cravings with its sweet licorice flavor
- Improves overall digestion and respiratory function

Aromatic Use
- Diffuse 3–4 drops. It also blends well with spicy scents like Cinnamon Bark and citrus oils like Lime.

Topical Use
- Apply 1–2 drops to 1 teaspoon of fractionated coconut oil and massage into your abdomen.
- Massage into tense areas.

GINGER (*Zingiber officinale*)
- Supports normal cortisol levels to minimize cravings and bingeing
- Reduces inflammation for better absorption of vitamins and nutrients
- Supports healthy digestion while reducing bloating and gas

Aromatic Use
- Diffuse 3 drops. Try adding 3 drops Wild Orange and 2 drops Ylang Ylang to boost energy and distract from afternoon cravings.

- Add 1 drop in the palm of your hand, rub together, and inhale.

Topical Use
- Dilute 1–2 drops with a carrier oil and massage over the lower abdomen.
- Dilute 1–2 drops with a carrier oil and massage where needed.

GRAPEFRUIT (*Citrus × paradisi*)

- Detoxifies and cleanses the body
- Inhibits water retention
- Minimizes bingeing and helps resist sugar cravings
- Supports a healthy metabolism
- Suppresses cravings

Aromatic Use
- Add 3–4 drops to a diffuser.

Topical Use
- Massage 1–2 drops with a carrier oil and apply directly into areas with excess fat deposits or create a soothing sugar scrub or body wash.
- Dilute with a carrier oil and massage into desired areas while breathing deeply.

WARNING: Avoid exposure to direct sunlight for at least 12 hours after applying topically, as citrus oils are phototoxic.

Internal Use
- Boost your morning smoothie by adding 1–2 drops.

LAVENDER (*Lavandula angustifolia*)

- Reduces feelings of stress, anxiety, and depression to reduce emotional eating
- Helps to lower cortisol levels
- Calms the mind and body for restful sleep

Aromatic Use
- Add a few drops to your pillow or bedclothes before bedtime.
- Dilute 15 drops in ¼ cup water in a 3-ounce glass spray bottle. Shake and spritz.

- Add 3–4 drops to a diffuser anytime you need to experience calm, and especially before bedtime.

Topical Use

- Apply 1–2 drops with a carrier oil to your soles and/or pulse points before bedtime.
- Add 4 drops to ½ cup Epsom salts and dissolve into warm bath.
- Add 10–15 drops to your DIY body wash.

LEMON (*Citrus limon*)

- Supresses cravings
- Detoxifies and cleanses the body
- Suppresses appetite to prevent overeating
- Aids in healthy digestion

Aromatic Use

- Diffuse 3–4 drops to cleanse your environment and suppress cravings. Combine with Lime, Lavender, or Rosemary.

Topical Use

- Add 4–5 drops to a handful of sugar or oatmeal and use as an exfoliating body scrub.

WARNING: Avoid direct exposure to sunlight for at least 12 hours, as citrus oils are phototoxic.

Internal Use

- Dilute 1 drop in 1 cup liquid and sip throughout the day.
- Add 1 drop to your morning green smoothies and water infusions.

PEPPERMINT (*Mentha piperita*)

- Decreases gas and bloating
- Reduces cravings by altering olfactory senses
- Suppresses appetite and cravings
- Boosts mood and awakens senses naturally

Aromatic Use

- Add 1 diluted drop to your palms, rub, and inhale deeply.

- Diffuse 2 drops with 2 drops Wild Orange and 2 drops Frankincense.
- Diffuse 2 drops with 3 drops Grapefruit.

Topical Use
- Dilute 1–2 drops with a carrier oil and massage into abdomen.
- Dilute 1–2 drops with a carrier oil and massage into tense areas and muscles.
- Combine 1–2 drops with 2 drops of Lavender and add to a carrier oil for a relaxing massage.
- Add 1 drop to your shampoo or conditioner and massage into scalp.

WARNING: The menthol content of Peppermint essential oil causes a cooling effect on the skin and can cause irritation if transferred to sensitive areas. Always dilute with a carrier oil if irritation occurs and NEVER try to wash the oil off. The water will repel the oil and drive it in deeper.

Cheryl's Story

Cheryl, age forty-eight, reached out to participate in the 14-Day Rescue Plan because she considered herself an emotional eater and she craved carbs, sugar, and diet soda on a daily basis. She desperately wanted to reset her eating habits and cravings. By the end of the 14-Day Rescue Plan Cheryl reported that all her cravings disappeared, especially her late-night carb cravings.

"I learned so much about why I have the cravings I have and how I can use essential oils to stop them in their tracks," she told me. "My go-to essential oil was Peppermint. It worked every time I struggled with late-night cravings, and the blend I still use each day is the Cut the Cravings Diffuser Blend (page 146). It gives me an energy boost and even helps to lift my mood."

Essential Oil Blends

Aromatic Diffuser Blends

Calm, Sweet Calm Diffuser Blend

3 drops Lavender essential oil
2 drops Lemon essential oil
2 drops Ginger essential oil

Wake Up and Focus Diffuser Blend

2 drops Bergamot essential oil
2 drops Lemon essential oil
1 drop Peppermint essential oil
1 drop Rosemary essential oil

Cut the Cravings Diffuser Blend

2 drops Cassia essential oil
2 drops Grapefruit essential oil
1 drop Peppermint essential oil
1 drop Ginger essential oil

Aromatic Personal Inhaler Blends

Energy Booster Inhaler Blend

8 drops Lemon essential oil
4 drops Ginger essential oil
3 drops Peppermint essential oil

Cravings Killer Inhaler Blend

3 drops Cinnamon Bark essential oil
5 drops Peppermint essential oil
5 drops Grapefruit essential oil

Sugar Banishing Inhaler Blend

5 drops Lavender essential oil
5 drops Lemon essential oil
3 drops Fennel essential oil
2 drops Dill essential oil

Topical Rollerball Blends

Crave-Control Rollerball Blend

Any time of day, any place, for any craving issue—this blend is the one to use. The power of Grapefruit and Peppermint to curb cravings will keep you focused, while Ginger will help to ease your digestive system and Cinnamon works to balance blood sugar levels. Immune support is an extra bonus to this blend, so roll it on!

10 drops Grapefruit essential oil
10 drops Peppermint essential oil
5 drops Cinnamon Bark essential oil
5 drops Ginger essential oil
Carrier oil of choice

Add the essential oils to a 10 mL glass rollerball bottle. Fill the rest of the way with your carrier oil and shake to blend oils. Replace the rollerball and top, and shake gently to combine. Roll on pulse points and deeply inhale.

Morning Craving-Buster Rollerball Blend

When sweet breakfast options beckon, use this blend to tame the sugar demons and carry on with your green smoothie preparations. This is especially helpful when you are dining out so that you can resist the menu temptations. It also contains a Peppermint/Wild Orange combo that will perk up your senses in the morning and keep you moving throughout the day.

10 drops Wild Orange essential oil
10 drops Peppermint essential oil
5 drops Neroli essential oil
Carrier oil of choice

Add the essential oils to a 10 mL glass rollerball bottle. Fill the rest of the way with a carrier oil. Replace the rollerball and top, and shake gently to combine. To use, simply roll on your pulse points and inhale deeply. Store tightly capped. This is a great blend to carry with you in your work bag or purse to ensure you are always ready to perk up and cut those cravings.

Sugar-Be-Gone Rollerball Blend

Peppermint and Citrus is an amazing combo that both curbs cravings and boosts your energy levels. When you start fantasizing about the vending machine or need to resist that luscious dessert option, roll this blend on your wrists and inhale deeply using your deep-breathing technique.

10 drops Peppermint essential oil
10 drops Grapefruit essential oil
10 drops Lemon essential oil
Carrier oil of choice

Add the essential oils to a 10 mL glass rollerball bottle and top off blend with a carrier oil of choice. Replace the rollerball and top, and shake gently to combine. Uncap and deeply inhale or apply to wrists.

Belly Bliss Rollerball Blend

During times when bloating and digestive discomfort begin to distract your focus, this blend will help with internal inflammation and rid your body of uncomfortable and often embarrassing side effects. Roll on your abdomen whenever your belly threatens harm, even if it is just from binge-eating or sugar overload.

8 drops Ginger essential oil
8 drops Fennel essential oil
6 drops Peppermint essential oil
Carrier oil of choice

Add the essential oils to a 10 mL glass rollerball bottle and top off blend with a carrier oil of choice. Replace the rollerball and top, and shake gently to combine. Apply directly on the abdomen, or apply to wrists and inhale.

Internal Uses

I'm always trying to come up with creative ways to get people to drink more water, as our bodies often mistake thirst for hunger. In order for our hormones to communicate with cell receptors, we need proper hydration, and that means following the 8 × 8 rule: eight 8-ounce glasses of water per day. I keep my water bottle with me at all times. The essential oils I use to boost my water also add powerful benefits to my overall health and wellness.

Thousands of women have had extraordinary success with my water infusions. In addition to reducing cravings, water infusions provide vitality, energy, and immune-boosting benefits.

As a rule of thumb, reach for your water first. Drink at the top of the hour and before meals. Let hydration combat your frustration!

Crave-Busting Water Infusion

1 grapefruit, sliced into wheels
1 drop Grapefruit essential oil
1 drop Peppermint essential oil
Ice cubes
1 quart filtered water

Layer the grapefruit in a large pitcher. Add the Grapefruit and Peppermint essential oils. Cover with ice (to your liking) and top with the water. Allow to steep for at least 30 minutes, but preferably for 2 to 3 hours, before serving.

Crave-Control Ice Cubes

½ cup lemon juice
1 drop Peppermint essential oil
3 cups filtered water

Combine the lemon juice, Peppermint, and water in a blender and blend until smooth, approximately 1 minute. Pour the mixture into ice cube trays and freeze. Add the cubes to a glass of water.

CHAPTER 9

Female Hormones: Fertility, Perimenopause, and Menopause

During their fertile years, women are celebrated for their ability to conceive and bear children, while infertility and loss are taboo or misunderstood topics. But they are not celebrated for their menstrual cycles—which are often the butt of jokes instead. Our society often forgets to honor women for the amazing creatures they are and the miracles their bodies can create.

In our Western culture, most of us are "taught" by the media to dread the onset of perimenopause, expecting to be burdened with hot flashes, irritability, mood swings, anxiety, depression, weight gain, insomnia, and more. Interestingly enough, other cultures in the world don't even have a word to describe menopause. They simply see it as a natural part of a woman's life transition, rather than a life-diminishing experience dominated by physical and mental symptoms. Actually, the symptoms that have become so negatively associated with menopause in our culture also don't exist in other places in the world. So I propose that we shift our perspective and celebrate this transitional time in our lives—a period from child-bearing years to wisdom-bearing years. We should admire our elders for their life experiences and learn from their struggles and successes. Getting to a place where this can happen is one of my hopes for our future as a society.

Changing your lifestyle to incorporate healthier habits of nutrition, exercise, stress management, and self-care rituals will serve to reset your body and mind and give you vivacity that you never knew was possible. Essential oils are key to this transformation. Proof of this came from a friend who had extremely bad PMS symptoms every month. I gently suggested that essential oils might help, but she just rolled her eyes. Finally, a month later, she called me in desperation and I whipped up the Monthly Massage Rollerball Blend (page 163) for her.

Soon, the phone rang, and she jumped right in with, "I really owe you an apology! I don't know what you put in that roller bottle, but it was like magic. I'm kicking myself for being so stubborn! I know that you said so, but why didn't you *tell me* that these oils worked so fast, and would make me feel so much better?"

I share stories like this because I know how difficult it can be to try something new, not knowing how it's going to work. Sometimes it can take years before we find the solution to a problem that truly transforms our health and well-being. This was also the case for my mom, one of my first success stories. She was already using essential oils, but not specifically for hormone support. Her hormone levels had been imbalanced all her adult life, but when she hit peri-menopause, she was not only physically miserable but also her sugar cravings became completely unmanageable. Every time I'd go over to her house, I'd find new hiding places where she'd stashed her favorite chocolate candy!

Her gynecologist prescribed bio-identical hormone replacement therapy (BHRT), which didn't relieve her symptoms; she found her-self feeling sadder and more tired throughout the day. Although I know that BHRT can work for some women, it was not the answer for my mother. She weaned herself off BHRT in favor of a lifestyle adjustment, and I put her on the 14-Day Rescue Plan, reworked her idea of exercise, ensured that her self-care rituals would calm her stress levels and support a restful night's sleep, and incorporated daily essential-oil support. In the course of only three months she lost thirty-five pounds, her hot flashes diminished and then vanished, the depression significantly improved, and her energy bounced back. Even more exciting for her, she was sleeping all the way through the night, a feat she hadn't accomplished in years. Her transformation was unique to her individual situation, just as yours will be.

The Why Behind Female Hormones

As discussed in Chapter 1, there are three stages for all women, each defined by a certain level of female hormones. During a woman's fertile years, from puberty until, usually, her late thirties or early forties, estrogen and progesterone are responsible for monthly men-struation or pregnancy. During perimenopause, which often takes a decade or more, female hormone levels begin a gradual decline. Estrogen levels fluctuate as the ovaries slack off production, and the menstrual cycle becomes erratic. Menopause arrives when a wom-an's period has completely ceased for a year.

The Most Common Symptoms of Perimenopause

Brain fog

Breast tenderness

Chest pain/palpitations

Fatigue/lethargy

Hair thinning, loss, and
dryness

Headaches/migraines

Hot flashes/night sweats

Libido (reduced)

Osteopenia (low bone
density)

PMS/irregular periods/
heavy flow/cramps

Skin issues: loss
of elasticity,
pigmentation, acne,
dryness

Sleeplessness/other
sleep problems

Urinary incontinence

Vaginal dryness/
thinning (painful
sex)

Weight gain, belly fat

Your Hormones for Reproduction

Debilitating PMS symptoms should not be a part of any woman's normal cycle. Instead, they're a sign that your reproductive hormones are out of balance. In addition, as estrogen levels naturally drop during perimenopause, the symptoms of perimenopause can eventually become crippling. Even though ovarian production of hormones slowly ceases, the adrenal glands continue to produce them, so any imbalance or stressor that affects the adrenals can throw hormones out of whack.

Estrogen

Produced primarily in the ovaries, "estrogen" is a general term used to describe any of the compounds producing estrus, such as estrone, estradiol, and estriol. They rule our reproductive systems by regulating menstrual cycles during our fertile years as well as directly affecting our growth and development.

Progesterone

Produced in the ovaries during menstruation, the placenta during pregnancy, and the adrenal glands, progesterone's role is to prepare the uterus for a viable pregnancy. If implantation doesn't occur during any given month, progesterone levels drop, causing a monthly period. If it does, the egg implants into the thickened lining of the uterus and progesterone production continues until the placenta takes over at around twelve weeks.

Testosterone

Not present only in a male's body, testosterone is also produced in the ovaries and adrenals of women in order to influence bone strength, muscle mass, and support a healthy libido.

Cortisol

As detailed in Chapter 5 and in nearly every other chapter, stress continues to be the biggest offender and catalyst for hormonal imbalance. Unfortunately, chronic stress directly influences the reproductive hormones. Symptoms begin to crop up: inner-tube weight gain, decreased muscle mass, binge-eating and cravings for sugar and unhealthy comfort food, irregular menstrual periods in fertile years, PMS, exhaustion, brain fog—basically everything that feeds into the stereotype of the "hysterical" woman on her monthly period.

Estrogen Dominance (Dysestrogenism)

The condition in which the body has too much estrogen and not enough progesterone to balance it out, estrogen dominance in my practice seems to be a full-blown epidemic. Many symptoms are attributed to it, but they're often the same ones that occur with other so-called women's issues such as PMS, perimenopause, and depression or anxiety disorders. Estrogen dominance can cause decreased libido, fatigue, bloating, and weight gain; prolonged high levels can cause more serious concerns such as fibroids in the breasts, ovarian cysts, endometriosis, infertility, and even some cancers, among others.

Cortisol can influence estrogen levels as well if too much of it leads to the shutdown of the reproductive system. Even more dangerous is when women are treated with HRT that contains both estrogen and progesterone, which has been shown to cause cortisol levels to rise at night. Add in xenoestrogens from toxins and the products we use, and we have more estrogen than the liver can properly metabolize. A low-fiber diet exacerbates this as your digestive system has trouble filtering out excess estrogen through regular bowel movements. Plus, if you've taken birth control pills, you may have created a dam full of synthetic estrogen just waiting to spill over, too.

In our modern environment, we all may be suffering from a bit of estrogen dominance. Other symptoms that we commonly attribute to normal living—allergies and asthma, sinus issues, headaches, arthritis, and even cancer development—might be attributed to it. The reality is that we need some major changes and overall awareness before we will see any real change in our health and wellness.

Understanding Birth Control and Hormone Replacement Therapy

In our fertile years, irregular periods or mood issues are often attributed to imbalanced hormones, and birth control pills full of synthetic hormones are prescribed. Many women then experience a regular period for the first time in their lives, and they think, "I'm cured! What a relief to have a regular period without intense bleeding or cramps! What a convenience to predict my cycle each month!"

"This is further from the truth." They don't realize the harm these synthetic hormones can do to their reproductive system and body in the process. Birth control is a *contraceptive*, not a hormone solution.

Anything synthetic that we add to our bodies raises a huge red flag for me, and it does for most functional practitioners and those following functional medicine practices. But in the Western world, we seem to be fine with recommending more synthetic hormones and not getting to the root cause of the problem.

Even more controversial is the trend to request bio-identical hormones rather than their synthetic counterparts, assuming that "bio-identical" means "natural" when it does not. BHRT has not been properly researched, so women wishing to start HRT and BHRT should always discuss the benefits and risks of treatment with their functional practitioner, taking into account their age, medical history, risk factors, and personal preferences.

Emotional Triggers

Hormonal imbalances can most definitely cause emotional upset and mood swings, but those aren't the emotional triggers I want to mention here. I'm more concerned with the damage that we do to ourselves when we pretend to be "normal" and power through our symptoms instead of dealing with root causes. We condition ourselves to think that what we are experiencing is normal for everyone, and we choose not to discuss our issues, even with our health-care providers.

Only we know our own truths and our own emotional triggers. I recommend keeping a journal where you can log your emotional timeline throughout the month. Do this for three months so you can begin to see patterns based on events in your life and the time of the month when they occur. Correlating recurring symptoms with a specific time frame while noting if there were any emotional triggers can help you to discover where you need some extra support.

How to Support Female Hormones with Essential Oils

No essential oil can stop the natural decline in hormonal levels that comes with age, as this is an unavoidable physiological process. As you know, essential oils are not hormones and cannot be used as hormones, but they can ease the way. Many symptoms during this transitional period can be alleviated with the potency and power of essential oils.

Most important, reducing chronic stress, revamping your diet and exercise routine, and ridding your environment of toxic chemicals and xenoestrogens will normalize your body as much as possible. This will help you to achieve this seemingly elusive hormonal balance, which actually looks more like an ebb and flow of fluctuating hormones that regulate themselves.

Preferred Essential Oils

CLARY SAGE (*Salvia sclarea*)
- Eases menstrual cramps and tension by relaxing smooth muscles
- Decreases the body's cortisol levels naturally
- Relaxes, soothes, and balances the mind and body

Aromatic Use
- Diffuse 3–4 drops at night.
- Diffuse 2 drops with 2 drops Lavender.

Topical Use
- Dilute 1–2 drops with a carrier oil and massage into abdomen during your menstrual cycle.
- Dilute 1–2 drops with a carrier oil and rub into your soles and pulse points.

LAVENDER (*Lavandula angustifolia*)

- Calms the mind and body to support a restful night's sleep
- Eases and calms feelings of anxiety, stress, and tension while rebalancing emotions
- Relieves discomfort associated with menstrual cycles

Aromatic Use

- Diffuse 3–4 drops.
- Add 1–2 drops to pillows and bedclothes before bedtime.

Topical Use

- Dilute 1–2 drops with a carrier oil and massage into the temples and the back of the neck.
- Add 3–4 drops to ½ cup Epsom salts and dissolve into a warm bath.

YLANG YLANG (*Cananga odorata*)

- Calming and uplifting scent that can boost your mood and relieve tension
- Reduces blood pressure and provides a total-body relaxation
- Offers daily support for hormonal balance, including boosting libido

Aromatic Use

- Diffuse 3–4 drops.

Topical Use

- Dilute 1–2 drops with a carrier oil and rub into wrists and the back of the neck.
- Dilute 1–2 drops with a carrier oil and massage into tense muscles.
- Add 3–4 drops to ½ cup Epsom salts and dissolve into a warm bath.

BERGAMOT (*Citrus bergamia*)

- Calms and soothes the mind and body while uplifting the mood during times of stress and tension
- Reduces heart rate and blood pressure to calm the body's stress responses

- Alleviates stress and anxiety to uplift your overall vitality and mood

Aromatic Use
- Diffuse 3–4 drops.

Topical Use
- Dilute 1–2 drops with a carrier oil and massage into abdomen during moments of stress or during your menstrual period.
- Dilute 1–2 drops with a carrier oil and apply to your soles.

THYME (*Thymus vulgaris*)

- Reduces high stress levels to promote and support a healthy immune system
- Supports the body during the hormonal transition into peri-menopause
- Provides powerful antioxidants to the body to support a healthy immune system

Aromatic Use
- Diffuse 3–4 drops.

Topical Use
- Dilute 1–2 drops with a carrier oil and massage into ankles and soles.

GERANIUM (*Pelargonium graveolens*)

- Supports emotional balance with its calming and grounding aroma
- Alleviates pent-up stress and soothes frazzled nerves
- Rejuvenates and revitalizes skin, complexion, and hair

Aromatic Use
- Diffuse 3–4 drops.
- Inhale directly from the bottle.

Topical Use
- Dilute 1–2 drops with a carrier oil and massage into the body where needed.
- Dilute 1–2 drops with a carrier oil and apply to skin post-shower.

Christine's Story

Christine was fifty-one years old, a registered nurse, and an avid gardener on the weekends, who came to me with severe hot flashes, exhaustion in the morning due to lack of sleep, and stubborn weight that she couldn't seem to lose, no matter how much she dieted. She was also getting headaches several times a week.

Christine was experiencing low levels of estrogen due to menopausal changes. **My recommendations were as follows:**

- An essential oil spray of Peppermint, Clary Sage, and Lavender anytime she felt a hot flash coming on.
- Peppermint, Lavender, and Frankincense essential oils for head and neck tension.
- Lavender and Vetiver in a spray for sleep, and Clary Sage and Cedarwood to the bottom of her feet and in her diffuser before going to bed.
- To reduce cravings, increased hydration with water with Lemon essential oil in the afternoon.
- Supplements: multivitamin, 300 mg magnesium glycinate, 40 mg black cohosh, 1000 mg maca in green smoothies, and a phytoestrogen complex.
- The 14-Day Rescue Plan to help reset her blood sugar levels and boost her metabolism.

Within three weeks, Christine experienced significantly fewer hot flashes and she was sleeping a solid seven hours each night. She lost seven pounds on the eating plan and she no longer needed to rely on sugar to get through her twelve-hour nursing shifts.

After two months, Christine told me she'd had only

three hot flashes and had lost seven more pounds. "I love that I am sleeping throughout the night and that I feel like I have more control over my metabolism and hormones," she said. "I can't believe how helpful essential oils were for my 4 p.m. cravings and for shutting off my brain."

Essential Oil Blends

Aromatic Diffuser Blends

Hormonal Support Diffuser Blend

2 drops Clary Sage essential oil
1 drop Geranium essential oil
1 drop Ylang Ylang essential oil

Emotional Unwind Diffuser Blend

2 drops Geranium essential oil
2 drops Lemongrass essential oil
2 drops Ylang Ylang essential oil

Uplift and Balance Diffuser Blend

2 drops Clary Sage essential oil
2 drops Grapefruit essential oil
4 drops Neroli essential oil

Aromatic Body Spray

Cool-It Body Spray

8 drops Clary Sage essential oil
6 drops Geranium essential oil
6 drops Peppermint essential oil
¼ cup witch hazel

In a 2-ounce glass spray bottle, add the essential oils and fill the rest of the way with witch hazel. Replace the spray top, shake to combine, and spritz onto neck, décolletage, and any area that heats up with hormonal stress.

Topical Rollerball Blends

Hormone Synergy Rollerball Blend

10 drops Clary Sage essential oil
7 drops Lavender essential oil
5 drops Geranium essential oil
4 drops Bergamot essential oil
4 drops Ylang Ylang essential oil
Carrier oil of choice

Add essential oils to a 10 mL glass rollerball bottle and fill the rest with the carrier oil. Replace the rollerball top and cap, then shake gently to blend. To use, roll on abdomen over ovaries and on your pulse points (behind ears, on wrists and ankles, and over heart) two or three times per day.

Monthly Massage Rollerball Blend

10 drops Lavender essential oil
8 drops Clary Sage essential oil
4 drops Roman Chamomile essential oil
4 drops Ylang Ylang essential oil
Carrier oil of choice

Add the essential oils to a 10 mL glass rollerball bottle and fill the rest with the carrier oil. Replace the rollerball top and cap, and then shake gently to blend. To use, roll over abdomen as needed.

Stress-Free Massage Rollerball Blend

10 drops Lavender essential oil
10 drops Clary Sage essential oil
5 drops Peppermint essential oil
Carrier oil of choice

Add the essential oils to a 10 mL glass rollerball bottle and fill the rest of the way with the carrier oil. Replace the rollerball top and cap, and shake gently to combine. To use, roll on your shoulders, temples, the back of your neck, and on your wrists and ankles and massage in slowly. Then cup your hands over your nose and breathe deeply.

Topical Bath Blends

Basic Bath Soak

8–10 drops essential oils of choice, or one of the blends below
   (suggested: Clary Sage, Frankincense, Lavender, Roman Chamomile, or Ylang Ylang)
1 cup sea salt
1 cup Epsom salts or magnesium flakes
½ cup high-quality baking soda

Add the essential oils to the dry ingredients and swirl into a warm bath to dissolve.

Relax and De-stress Bath Blend

3 drops Lavender essential oil
3 drops Cedarwood essential oil
2 drops Clary Sage essential oil

PMS Relief Bath Blend

2 drops Clary Sage essential oil
1 drop Roman Chamomile essential oil
1 drop Geranium essential oil
1 drop Lavender essential oil

Supplements to Support Female Hormones

Supplementation can be particularly helpful in support of female hormone levels, especially if you are taking the right ones, so be sure to discuss them with your trusted health-care provider. While you may not need to take these supplements indefinitely, I recommend trying the ones you need for at least three months to see how your body improves, and then discuss continued usage with your health-care provider. For a complete list of hormone supplements and how to make over your hormone medicine cabinet, go to www.drmariza .com/supplements.

Ashwagandha + *Rhodiola Rosea.* The combination of these two herbs has been proven to help boost energy while strongly supporting adrenal function and combating fatigue. As adaptogenic herbs, they can help your body to fight stressors naturally while their rejuvenating properties can revitalize your body and mind. They have numerous other benefits to your overall wellness, including immune support, fat-burning power, and hormonal and overall balance.

B-Complex Vitamins (B_1, B_2, B_3, B_6, B_{12}). These are essential for all vital functions, for the health of our sexual organs, and as essential players in libido levels, especially post-menopausal. By supporting the adrenal production of sex hormones and keeping a healthy hormonal production, B-complex vitamins reduce symptoms associated with hormonal flux, including headaches, fatigue, PMS, and vaginal dryness.

Black Cohosh (*Cimicifuga racemosa*). This is a member of the buttercup family used by Native Americans to aid in childbirth and support symptoms related to the female reproductive system. Research has shown it to influence the serotonin receptors, effectively alleviating hot flashes and balancing mood. Though classified as a phytoestrogen, its estrogenic effects on the body are nil, making black cohosh one of the most popular supplements related to PMS and menopause owing to its safety and efficacy. It may also help to prevent a range of women's cancers. It has been used in Germany since the 1940s under the name Remifemin. Research now suggests that it is most effective when used only for a prescribed six-month time period rather than long term to avoid potential side effects.

Chasteberry (*Vitex agnus-castus*). This plant grows in the Mediterranean and has been used for centuries to promote fertility and libido by increasing progesterone levels. It is believed to affect the pituitary gland's release of luteinizing hormone (LH), lowers prolactin that affects menstrual cycles, and affects several different neurotransmitters. Although we don't know precisely *how* it works, we know that it *does* work and is prescribed in more nontraditional medical practice for fertility issues related to low progesterone; it's also widely used in Germany for PMS and menstrual issues. It works well with black cohosh in improving emotional issues and hot flashes for both perimenopausal and postmenopausal women.

Magnesium glycinate. A crucial component in our bodies, it's a building block for DNA and is essential for proper functioning of the nervous, muscular, reproductive, and cardiovascular systems. It also supports the HPA axis by maintaining healthy cortisol levels and protecting your body from toxins and free radicals. In turn, this helps to amp up your libido and promote fertility for a healthy reproductive system. Magnesium greatly helps to alleviate symptoms from reproductive imbalances, such as PMS. The recommended dosage is 310–400 mg.

DIM (Diindolemethane). This is a phytochemical found in cruciferous vegetables that has been proven to reduce risk for breast, cervical, and other cancers influenced by estrogen. By increasing production of healthy estrogen and decreasing the bad, it can also alleviate symptoms of PMS, perimenopause, and menopause. It supports a healthy metabolism and aids the body in using female hormones as well as supporting healthy adrenal function.

Hops (*Humulus lupulus L.*). The female flowers of the hops plant, used to make beer, are also beneficial for female hormones—but you need to take this in a capsule, not as the alcoholic beverage! Hops contain 8-prenylnaringenin, a super-potent phytoestrogen. I don't recommend hops for everyone, especially since estrogen dominance is so common, but during perimenopause and menopause, when estrogen levels drop, it can be helpful when regulated by your health-care provider. It has been shown to reduce the vasomotor symptoms of menopause, such as hot flashes, insomnia, and fatigue. By simulating estrogen, hops help to stimulate progesterone production as well. It has also been shown to assist nursing mothers in the production of prolactin, which helps stimulate milk production.

Maca (*Lepidium meyenii*). Though referred to as an herb, maca is actually a root common to the Peruvian Andes and is eaten there. Taken as a supplement, it has been found to greatly support the symptoms of PMS, balance hormones, and support healthy reproductive function, as well as being a well-known aphrodisiac.

Self-Care Rituals for Female Hormones

Here are some easy ways to balance your hormones, whether your period has arrived or if you're going through perimenopause.

Monthly Clean-Out Ritual

Owing to the overwhelming impact of xenoestrogens and toxins in our environment, I recommend doing a monthly clean-out of your kitchen, cleaning cabinet, and personal-care and beauty products. I always clean one cabinet or drawer the last day of the month so that when the next month starts, I can start fresh with new hope. Chapter 14 has many more details about what to do.

De-Stress Ritual

Try to do a couple of the rituals suggested in Chapter 5 if you haven't already begun to incorporate them into your repertoire. I highly recommend finding a spiritual practice that speaks to you as well, as the benefits greatly differentiate an empowered woman from an overwhelmed woman.

Stop and Breathe Ritual

Try to start and end each day with a deep-breathing ritual. As soon as you wake up, do ten deep-belly breaths. Close your eyes and focus on something that makes you truly happy. This sends the message to your body that you are in control and stress is managed. Add this ritual to mid-morning, lunchtime, mid-afternoon, and dinnertime, and before long, it will be second nature. Or, set your alarm for every three hours as a reminder, or add it before you eat. This is a great ritual allowing you to work the stress out whenever you need to in the future.

Nurture Your Skin Ritual

As the largest organ of your body, your skin needs some extra love on a daily basis, especially from massages, bath soaks, deep mois-ture treatments, essential-oil shower treatments, and essential-oil steam facials. One of my favorites is dry brushing, which improves circulation, stimulates the lymphatic system, helps get rid of toxins (like those pesky xenoestrogens), and gets the skin glowing again.

Deep Essential Oil Ritual

If you're having cramps, harboring tension, feeling muscle aches, or experiencing any other sort of internal discomfort, an amazing way to get the essential oils and blends deep into your system while sup-porting relaxation is to use a warm-water compress. A warm, wet washcloth placed on top of wherever you massaged in essential oils will push them deeper into your body and simultaneously create an aromatherapeutic experience for your environment.

CHAPTER 10

Libido

Are you blushing yet? Because I am. Let's talk about sex . . . or lack thereof.

I struggled with low libido because of a hormonal imbalance from a very early age. It started when I went on birth control pills when I was eighteen. I assumed my low libido was normal and I tried to make myself enjoy sex. But it was painful. It was anything but sexy. Honestly, for years I thought I was broken. I was so embarrassed, ashamed, overwhelmed, and alone. I mean, who do you talk to about this? Your mom? Your friends? Definitely *not* your boyfriend or your partner. I just kept it to myself, pushed forward in my chaotic life, and pretended I was sexually fulfilled when I wasn't.

What I didn't realize then was that my loss of libido came primarily from hormonal imbalance and birth control. Yes, there are other reasons women may experience a decrease in libido, such as illness or medications, but for most women it's hormonal. That means not even the best relationship and most understanding partner can fix it. Hormones, baby. It's *hormones*.

Does that mean that relationships aren't players in libido issues? Absolutely not. Sexual energy between two partners, as well as their intimacy levels and ability to connect on an emotional level, strongly support libido and healthy sexual function. Strong relationships enable you to work on fixing the problem, and you should be able to communicate with your partner about why you might not be ready to jump into bed at any given moment. Thankfully, life blessed me with an amazing man to share my world with, and I experienced an intimacy with him that allowed me to be open about my libido.

Our society's view of the female libido is long overdue for an overhaul, as well. Movies and TV shows perpetuate the stereotypes of women as either frigid and prudish or sexual wildcats unable to satisfy promiscuous desires. Men, on the other hand, get to be the sexy, romantic Casanovas who sweep women off their feet with their irresistible pheromones and charming sweet talk. Their problem seems to be libido overdrive. None of this is true in real life, of course, and it's about time for women to understand that hormonal issues affect the majority of us in this world—even men. *You are not alone.*

Sex is one of the greatest delights we can have. Having sex reduces chronic stress and helps you sleep. It's anti-aging. It burns calories. It's fun. It connects you in the most intimate way to your partner. There should always be joy and awesomeness with it. There's no reason not to be fulfilled, and essential oils can help you move from lack of libido to a healthy sex life.

The Why *Behind a Loss of Libido*

Along with their female hormones, women have much lower levels of male hormones, called *androgens*. The primary androgen is testosterone, and, not surprisingly, it plays a large role in your libido levels—especially as it begins to decline in our mid-twenties rather than waiting for that perimenopausal swing a decade or so later. Add in the trauma our bodies face from the chronic stress that shuts down our reproductive system in favor of survival, and this can become a real problem. Estrogen dominance or testosterone dominance can cause issues like polycystic ovarian syndrome, adrenal fatigue, thyroid issues, medications, alcohol and smoking, and exhaustion can also contribute to the decline of a healthy libido.

By the time perimenopause does roll around, women are often already dealing with low libido and suffering silently, mourning its loss while doing little to remedy the situation because they think it's a lost cause, or have been told again that it's just life. But it's not!

Studies have shown that the biggest complaint among perimenopausal and menopausal women is lack of libido, vaginal dryness, and inability to orgasm. If you continue to ignore the signs and symptoms of hormonal imbalance, you're missing an opportunity to be proactive about your own health. It's time to take back control of your health.

Your Hormones for Libido

Cortisol

Stress causes the body to go into survival mode and send the signal that it's not a good time for intimacy. An out-of-balance reproductive system that isn't producing the proper amounts of estrogen and testosterone to support a healthy libido leaves the sex drive by the wayside in favor of survival.

Estrogen

When an imbalance in progesterone levels develops, many symptoms can arise, as was discussed in Chapter 9. Low libido and vaginal dryness are two of them.

Testosterone

Normal testosterone levels trigger the hypothalamus to prepare your erogenous zones for sexual activity. Half the testosterone in the body is produced by the androgens, DHEA and androstene-dione; the adrenals and ovaries are responsible for their release. During perimenopause, however, testosterone levels have already declined by half, and this decline continues into menopause along with lowered adrenal production and estrogen levels. The ovaries still produce testosterone, but less of it, and when levels are low, libido is low as well.

The biggest problem women face with testosterone is when they are also taking oral contraceptives. The pill increases globulin levels, which attracts free testosterone available in the body—poaching the testosterone that our bodies need and resulting in decreased libido, vaginal dryness, and uncomfortable sexual activity. If you are on the pill, I highly suggest discussing alternatives with a trusted health-care professional.

Emotional Triggers

While hormones play a powerful role in libido, your emotions can also cause your libido to suffer. Many of my patients have allowed themselves to suffer with unsatisfying sex, but felt obligated to please their partners no matter how traumatic or painful it felt. Some even admit that once they get into the act, the renewal of intimacy enabled them to enjoy the experience, but the initial step can be the hardest hurdle to overcome. But, more often than not, I have seen them literally condition themselves to have an adverse reaction to sex owing to their negative experiences with low libido and sex in general.

Body issues may also cause women to feel ashamed, nervous, or just plain unsexy. Weight changes, wrinkles, sagging, and childbirth can trigger a lot of anxiety. When you're no longer comfortable in your own skin, and feeling unable to be vulnerable and honest with your partner, every attempt at intimacy can feel like the very first time.

Fear may also be an issue, since many women find themselves too nervous to truly ask for what they want or guide their partner to help them reach orgasm. Some women lack the basic understanding of anatomy in order to understand where their pleasure zones are, while others have a misconception of how sex should be performed. Sex education classes in school, coupled with unrealistic depictions of sex in the media (and in pornography), have left a huge gap in understanding as well. Most of us know how *not* to get pregnant and what's supposed to happen once intercourse begins, but the middle ground—the priming and foreplay—are what's missing. Sometimes it's easier to say no rather than working with your partner to have a satisfying sex life.

You should never feel pressured or guilty for not wanting to have sex. There are plenty of alternatives to the actual act of intercourse, such as foreplay, cuddling, massage, and other intimate acts. I recommend exploring these with your partner to build trust and intimacy, and maybe even to discover or rediscover what each of you finds pleasurable in working toward the natural moment when intercourse may be the next step. Getting your body primed for the act, making sure that natural lubrication is happening, and being sure that you both feel comfortable moving to the next step are all about communication, understanding, and respect.

Regardless of your libido, your emotional state can greatly affect your sexual satisfaction. Essential oils can help you be comfortable, relaxed, and turned on enough. But before that can happen, you need to address any hormonal issues that may be hampering your success.

How to Support Your Libido with Essential Oils

With their powerful, aromatic properties that immediately affect the limbic brain, connecting into your pleasure centers so that you're able to relax and be open to sexual pleasure, essential oils are an ideal solution for libido issues. By stimulating the pituitary, the master gland for hormone production, they also help ensure that the hormones you need for a proper sex drive are triggered.

Everyone deserves to enjoy sex. Craving it, relishing it, desiring it—these are all normal sensations. Learning to express your desires and communicate intimately with your partner are all positive steps toward reviving the emotional side of your libido. I want you to stop feeling like sex is an obligation and start seeing it as a life-affirming, pleasurable, intimacy-enhancing adventure.

For centuries, essential oils have been used to promote relaxation and increase sensuality. They are able to evoke a feeling of eroticism that can make you feel truly sexy. Inhaling them and applying them is like adorning yourself in something truly beautiful. And they *work*.

Preferred Essential Oils

CLARY SAGE (*Salvia sclarea*)

- Relaxes and soothes the mind and body while balancing your mood
- Helps to relieve stress and calm your mind and body
- Commonly used to stimulate sexual energy and boost libido

Aromatic Use

- Diffuse 3–4 drops.
- Inhale directly from the bottle and practice deep breathing.

Topical Use

- Apply 1–2 drops with a carrier oil to pulse points and wear as a perfume throughout the day or before intimacy.
- Add 2–3 drops to ½ cup Epsom salts dissolved in a warm bath. Add Geranium or Jasmine for an extra libido boost.
- Dilute 1–2 drops with your favorite carrier oil and use as a deep massage prior to intimacy.

GERANIUM (*Pelargonium graveolens*)

- Calms and grounds emotions while naturally reducing stress
- Elevates feelings of happiness and love while relaxing the mind and body

Aromatic Use

- Diffuse 3–4 drops.
- Add 10 drops to a 2-ounce spray bottle and spritz bedclothes to prepare for intimacy.

Topical Use

- Dilute 1–2 drops with your favorite carrier oil and use as a massage.
- Apply after a warm bath or shower by diluting 1 part oil and 1 part carrier oil, then massaging into skin.

JASMINE (*Jasminum grandiflorum*)

- Soothes and calms the mind and body
- Boosts confidence and enhances feelings of sensuality and arousal
- Eases fatigue and boosts mood to bring optimism and zap fears

Aromatic Use

- Diffuse 3–4 drops before an intimate evening.
- Add 10–15 drops to a 2-ounce glass spray bottle of water and spritz bedclothes before intimacy.

Topical Use

- Dilute 1–2 drops with your favorite carrier oil and apply to pulse points.
- Dilute 1–2 drops with your favorite carrier oil and apply to your soles.

NEROLI (*Citrus x aurantium*)

- Encourages sexual desire and reduces inhibitions
- Relieves symptoms associated with menopause
- Calms the mind and body and reduces anxiety and stress

Aromatic Use

- Inhale directly from the bottle while practicing deep breathing.
- Apply to palms, rub together, cup over nose, and inhale deeply several times.

Topical Use

- Dilute 1–2 drops with your favorite carrier oil and use as a sensual massage. Add Lavender or Ylang Ylang for a more intense experience.
- Dilute 1–2 drops with your favorite carrier oil and apply to pulse points.

ROSE (*Rosa damascena*)

- Uplifts emotions and alleviates feelings of depression
- Known historically as a stimulating and intoxicating aphrodisiac

Aromatic Use

- Diffuse 2–3 drops.
- Add 5 drops to a 2-ounce glass spray bottle of water and spritz on bedclothes prior to intimacy.

Topical Use

- Dilute 1–2 drops with your favorite carrier oil and apply to pulse points, especially over heart.
- Add 1–2 drops to ½ cup Epsom salts and dissolve in a warm bath. Soak alone or with your partner.

SANDALWOOD (*Santalum album*)

- Prized for its ability to act as an aphrodisiac for men and women
- Balances hormonal issues while improving mood
- Relieves anxiety associated with intimacy

Aromatic Use

- Diffuse 2–3 drops.
- Add 1 drop to pillows or bedclothes.

Topical Use

- Dilute 1–2 drops with your favorite carrier oil and apply to pulse points.
- Dilute 1–2 drops with your favorite carrier oil and use as a sensual massage.

YLANG YLANG (*Cananga odorata*)

- Enhances sensuality and boosts libido with aphrodisiac powers
- Calms emotions while increasing intimate energy

Aromatic Use

- Diffuse 3–4 drops.
- Add 10 drops to a 2-ounce glass spray bottle and spritz around the bedroom and on bedclothes.

Topical Use

- Add 2–3 drops to ½ cup Epsom salts and dissolve in a warm bath.
- Dilute 1–2 drops with your favorite carrier oil and massage into tense muscles.

Shellie's Story

Shellie, a forty-three-year-old fifth-grade teacher and mother of two children in college, came to me with concerns about PMS symptoms. She was regularly bloated close to the onset of her menstrual cycle and her periods were heavier than normal. She had no energy to work out after a long day with her students and she struggled with mood swings. Her lack of libido and erratic emotions had a detrimental effect on her relationship with her husband.

Shellie exhibited symptoms of low progesterone and chronic stress. **My recommendations were as follows:**

- Stress essential oil blend (with Clary Sage, Lavender, and Bergamot) and meditation three days a week to reduce the stress that was having an adverse effect on her hormone levels.
- Using Grapefruit and Ginger essential oils for energy and cravings in the afternoon.

- Using a Spice It Up Massage Blend (Sandalwood, Neroli, and Ylang Ylang) for an intimate massage once a week.
- Reducing sugar intake by focusing on savory meals, especially for breakfast and snacks.
- Substituting matcha lattes or yerba mate tea for coffee.
- Supplements: 500 mg of chasteberry, B-complex vitamin, 1500 mg maca in green smoothies, 600 mg of calcium citrate, and 300 mg of magnesium glycinate to support mood, hormone levels, and increase energy.
- Self-care rituals were a massage with aromatherapy twice a month, and a nighttime ritual with relaxing baths and diffusing essential oils to help her get into the mood for sex.

Within four weeks, Shellie experienced less bloating and mood swings before her period. Her weight stabilized during her luteal phase (before her menstrual cycle). She had more energy so she could work out thirty minutes a day, three times a week. She even lost five pounds. When I asked her about self-care rituals, she replied, "The rituals are the biggest blessing in my life. I feel more calm throughout the day and can handle stressful moments with grace. I am spending more time with my husband and we are both loving how essential oils are helping us to create more intimacy."

Essential Oil Blends

Aromatic Diffuser Blends

Simply Soothing Diffuser Blend

2 drops Neroli essential oil
2 drops Jasmine essential oil
2 drops Ylang Ylang essential oil

Get in the Mood Diffuser Blend

2 drops Neroli essential oil
2 drops Lavender essential oil
1 drop Sandalwood essential oil
1 drop Ylang Ylang essential oil

Excited Night Diffuser Blend

2 drops Sandalwood essential oil
2 drops Clary Sage essential oil
2 drops Geranium essential oil

Aromatic Room Spray

Turn Me On Room Spray

6 drops Sandalwood essential oil
4 drops Ylang Ylang essential oil
3 drops Geranium essential oil
2 drops Neroli essential oil
¼ cup distilled water

Add the essential oils to a 2-ounce glass spray bottle and fill with water. Cap and shake to blend before each use. Shake and spritz on pillows, comforters, and in the air before bed.

Topical Rollerball Blends

Passion Rollerball Blend

10 drops Clary Sage essential oil
8 drops Ylang Ylang essential oil
5 drops Neroli or Rose essential oil
Carrier oil of choice

Add the essential oils to a 10 mL glass rollerball bottle and fill with carrier oil of your choice. Replace the rollerball top and cap, and shake gently to combine. Apply to pulse points and over heart to enhance sensuality and get you in the mood for intimacy.

Sensual Sensation Rollerball Blend

3 drops Sandalwood essential oil
3 drops Geranium essential oil
3 drops Ylang Ylang essential oil
3 drops Clary Sage essential oil
Carrier oil of choice

Add the essential oils to a 10 mL glass rollerball bottle and fill with the carrier oil of your choice. Replace the rollerball top and cap, and shake gently to combine. Apply to pulse points and over heart.

Love Potion Rollerball Blend

6 drops Jasmine essential oil
6 drops Rose essential oil
6 drops Ylang Ylang essential oil
Carrier oil of choice

Add the essential oils to a 10 mL glass rollerball bottle and fill with the carrier oil of your choice. Replace the rollerball top and cap, and shake gently to combine. Apply to pulse points, especially behind the ears and down décolletage.

Topical Massage Blends

Sensual Touch Massage Blend

3 drops Ylang Ylang essential oil
2 drops Jasmine essential oil

Add essential oil recipe to 1 teaspoon jojoba, sweet almond, or fractionated coconut oil and gently massage into skin.

Thigh-High Massage Blend

2 drops Clary Sage essential oil
2 drops Lavender essential oil
1 drop Ylang Ylang essential oil

Add essential oil recipe to 1 teaspoon jojoba, sweet almond, or fractionated coconut oil and gently massage into skin.

Spice It Up Massage Blend

2 drops Sandalwood essential oil
1 drop Cinnamon essential oil
2 drops Wild Orange essential oil

Add essential oil recipe to 1 teaspoon jojoba, sweet almond, or fractionated coconut oil and gently massage into skin.

Shower and Bath Blend

Romantic Couples Bath Blend

¼ cup Epsom salts
2 drops Clary Sage essential oil
2 drops Geranium essential oil
1 drop Ylang Ylang essential oil

Dissolve the Epsom salts in a warm bath and then add the essential oils.

Self-Care Rituals for Libido

Remember that everyone is different and will therefore need to explore different self-care rituals—so it probably won't be as easy as just picking one from the list and expecting it to work instant wonders. Persistence and consistency are key. Don't give up! You're worth it!

Just Breathe Ritual

One of my favorite rituals for increasing libido is actually one of the easiest. Just breathe. Choose your favorite calming, anti-anxiety, or de-stressing essential oil and practice the deep-breathing technique. You will be one step closer to moving into a ritual aimed at arousal or balancing your emotions so that you can allow yourself to unwind and relax into pleasure.

Thigh-High Ylang Ylang Ritual

I was talking to my mom about essential oils and libido, and it prompted her to wink and share this with me, "Just put Ylang Ylang on your Ylang Ylang." I began laughing at her suggestion, because we both know that Ylang Ylang can play a vital role in boosting libido.

Whenever aphrodisiacs are mentioned, Ylang Ylang comes to mind, as its gorgeous yellow flower has been used to adorn wedding ceremonies and prepare newlyweds' bedchambers for that first night. A simple evening ritual or pre-intimacy ritual involves diluting Ylang Ylang with an equal amount of a carrier oil, and focusing on massaging it into your inner thighs. Begin knee level and work your way up with slow, circular motions, closing your eyes as you go and inhaling the intoxicating aroma as you focus on the object of your desire. Once you become more comfortable with this ritual, you can invite your partner to participate for a next-level sensual experience.

Sensual Massage Ritual

For most of us, human touch elicits warmth and a feeling of comfort as our bodies release oxytocin, the cuddle hormone. As skin is your largest organ, no wonder it can trigger powerful emotional and physical responses. Massage can also help you release fears and deep anxiety around intimacy.

I recommend experimenting with some of the single oils before moving on to one of the blends in this chapter. You can begin alone, finding your most tense spots, and use the aromatic scents to help you unwind. Eventually, invite your partner to join in the fun, with a low-expectation understanding that your sole aim is to provide or receive a massage—nothing more.

Also, it's important to know that sometimes essential oil massage can cause an emotional release, so you may find yourself weepy and more emotional. Don't be scared—it's a good thing to release pent-up emotions and get your body reset and balanced. I like to write down my reactions to essential oils when trying something new or when they elicit a different response from what I expected. Keep a small journal to track your usage so that you can record your emotional response to specific oils.

Dark Chocolate Meditation Ritual

Though many people like to wind down at night, or try to get themselves in the mood with a glass of wine, it can actually have the opposite effect on your libido. Inhibiting your emotional and physical response time doesn't allow you to be truly present in the moment to connect with your partner. Even worse, alcohol can be dehydrating, impede lubrication, and lower your testosterone levels, preventing you from climaxing.

But dark chocolate can slowly melt in your mouth as you meditate and focus on the sensuality of the silkiness on your palate and amp up your readiness. Known as an aphrodisiac, dark chocolate boasts two specific compounds that aid in getting you in the mood:

phenethylamine and tryptophan. *Phenethylamine* is the same compound released in the brain when people fall in love, while *tryptophan* is a precursor to serotonin, the brain chemical associated with happy moods and sexual arousal. Allow the flavor to penetrate your palate, stimulate your mood, and uplift your emotions while you focus on the happiness associated with sexual intimacy.

Private Time Ritual

Though it may seem ridiculous at first, you may need to schedule some time for yourself. Pick a time each week to have personal time so that you can focus on improving your sexual energy and libido. At first, this can be time spent solo, so that you can focus on your wants and needs, and discover if you have any emotional fears or perceived physical limitations that would keep you from enjoying intimacy. Use the essential oils to ease the way and to support your emotional and physical health.

Next, invite your partner to participate by making a standing date. Try to make it exclusive and private for the two of you, meaning it might be time to hire a babysitter! Unplug from technology, lock your doors, and check your inhibitions at the bedroom door.

This is an incredibly important thing for any super-busy and overwhelmed couple to stay on track. I know from experience, because sometimes I'm that person. I have to schedule a date with my husband, or we're so busy that it's just not going to happen. Trust me. Private time = intimate time = sexy time!

Yoga Ritual

If you find that intense physical training just isn't for you, or if you want to supplement your normal workout with something slower, I highly recommend adopting this yoga ritual. You can support your practice with a number of essential oils; try diffusing them during yoga and applying them to pulse points before and afterward. In addition, there are several poses that can support a woman's body and aid in the strengthening and flexibility of muscles needed during intimacy:

- To ease pent-up tension in your hip flexors while increasing flexibility, try the Pigeon Pose and/or Lizard pose.
- To strengthen your pelvic floor and improve orgasmic muscles, try the Bridge pose.
- To put you in the mindset for intimacy and stretch the entire body while releasing stress, try the staple yoga pose Downward Dog.
- To alleviate symptoms of menopause, try Goddess pose.
- To improve circulation and stimulate the ovaries while training your body for strength during intercourse, try Bound Angle pose.

CHAPTER 11

Emotions: Balancing Anxiety, Depression, and Mood Swings

Women are twice as likely as men to be diagnosed with a mood disorder. Although it's not fully clear why, I have a theory, based on the patients I've treated over the years. When women take on the weight of the world and try to be everything for everyone, we set ourselves up for disaster. Chronic stress leads to imbalanced hormones, which is coupled with lifestyle choices and neglect, and this becomes the foundation on which we attempt to thrive. It just isn't working.

Self-care *must* be a priority in our lives. If we don't take care of ourselves, how can we give the best of ourselves to everyone who depends on us? Being diagnosed with a mood disorder and being prescribed antidepressants may not help you rebuild the foundation you need to thrive in this modern world.

One of the most researched areas of aromatherapy is the effect essential oils have on emotions and mood, so we know that they can provide the support we need to achieve emotional success. If there's one thing I've learned, it's that being able to manage your feelings is key to having a happy and successful life. There is no magic bullet to heal emotional distress, as we all know. But there's also no reason for medical professionals to dispense antidepressants and other mood-altering medications *before* assessing whether or not their patients actually need them.

So many women have come to me precisely because they don't want to take antidepressants; they're frustrated and fed up with the side effects. They want a natural solution instead. They ask me if essential oils can cure a mood disorder, and I tell them that, no, they can't—but they certainly can help the journey to healing. A *lot*. Especially if what we are dealing with isn't actually a mood disorder but, rather, an imbalance of hormones caused by a combination of factors such as long-term stress, perimenopause, gut health, and lifestyle choices. If your hormones are out of whack and have contributed to feelings of depression and anxiety, balancing your hormones can also alleviate the feeling of being overwhelmed that is associated with emotional distress.

The Why Behind Emotions

In my practice, I have found three main causes for emotional distress: stress, lack of sleep, and hormonal imbalance. The most important thing to remember is that maintaining a healthy balance between neurotransmitters and hormones keeps our emotions and mood balanced as well. This is achieved with a foundation of diet and nutrition, exercise, and stress management, as well as healthy sleep routines and reduced toxic load. Essential oils help balance the emotions and mood, as well as other systems.

In particular, *chronic stress* causes cortisol levels to rise. When left unchecked, it creates feelings of being overwhelmed and worries can surface, impacting how we respond to our environment. Chronic stress also shuts down the digestive system, and since most of our serotonin is produced in the gut, the body's second brain, any disruption will undoubtedly play a role in our emotional well-being.

Your Hormones for Emotions

You already know that certain kinds of moods or emotions can be hormonally driven, especially during specific times of your menstrual cycle, or when your female hormones are in decline during perimenopause and menopause. Remember that we all have different genetic makeups, past experiences, personalities, and lifestyles; our moods are directly related to these factors, as well as psychosocial factors, environmental effects, and physiological makeup. There is no one fix for all of us, but learning to understand your body's signals will help you shift to a lifestyle that supports your hormones, especially when you use essential oils.

These hormones play a key role in your moods:

Estrogen. Because estrogen fluctuates with the menstrual cycle, it also influences mood, depending on where you are in your cycle. It also can increase serotonin levels while balancing it and other neurotransmitters.

Progesterone. As long as progesterone levels are in balance with estrogen levels, your mood shouldn't suffer. Progesterone has a calming effect that can ease anxiety or depression.

The Three Ps: PMS, PMDD, and Perimenopause

While PMS is often described as a mood-altering period during your monthly cycle, its symptoms can vary from slight to intense depending on the overall state of your body. Anything that happens right before your period can be considered part of typical PMS. Most women assume that some symptoms—cramps, headaches, tender breasts—are just normal to their cycle, and they focus on the mood issues as the major factor. Mood swings can vary from mild irritability and anxiety to full-blown depression, panic attacks, and severe rage. Snarky comments about PMS may compound the situation with a heavy dose of guilt and self-loathing. You need to rebalance your body as soon as possible or you may find that your perimenopausal years will be even more difficult.

PMDD, or premenstrual dysphoric disorder, leaves women in a state of debilitating depression and causes mood issues on a monthly basis. Severe sensations of hopelessness and of feeling overwhelmed, wild mood swings, uncontrollable irritability and even rage, and extreme anxiety and tension that disrupt women's normal activities are all characteristics of PMDD. As with the other hormonal issues, I have found that my patients benefit from a lifestyle reset when suffering these debilitating symptoms. Proper diet, nutrition, exercise, stress management, and sleep can do wonders for your overall system and help the body to heal itself. Essential oils can be the key to making this transformational change.

During perimenopause, your estrogen and progesterone levels decline, causing a hormonal imbalance that can trigger panic attacks, mood swings, feelings of worry, and depression. Ignoring these symptoms may cause them to linger when you enter menopause. Instead, connect with your health-care provider, and explore natural options to boost your emotional well-being. A lifestyle reset, some self-care, and essential oils are foundational components for supporting your emotional well-being!

Cortisol. You already know what too much cortisol does to the body. Chronic worry, stress, and anxiety can chisel away at us until we become a fraction of what we could be. Factor in traumatic events, or emotionally taxing illnesses, and it's no wonder we find ourselves feeling overwhelmed.

The Science Behind the Scents

There are three main ways essential oils can affect your emotions, depending on their primary constituents: uplifting/energizing, calming/soothing, and grounding/balancing. To appease my inner science nerd, let me speak a bit about the chemical composition that makes these essential oils the amazing tools they are for influencing mood.

Monoterpenes such as limonene, alpha-pinene, terpinene, and cymene powerfully affect mood by cleansing and stimulating emotion. Under the monoterpene umbrella of limonene are soothing essential oils like Black Pepper, Spearmint, and Dill, as well as uplifting citrus oils such as Bergamot, Wild Orange, Tangerine, Grapefruit, Lemon, and Lime. Alpha-pinenes are known for their restorative powers, including Frankincense, Juniper Berry, Helichrysum, Cypress, and Rosemary.

Sesquiterpenes such as caryophyllene, zingiberene, and alpha-cedrene do wonders for soothing the emotions, as they promote balance and mental clarity. The caryophyllene found in Vetiver, Copaiba, Melissa, and Ylang Ylang soothes frazzled emotions, as do the zingiberene found in Ginger and the alpha-cedrene in Cedarwood.

Alcohols such as santalol, linalool, geraniol, and menthol fall into the categories of clarifying, calming, energizing, and stabilizing, as they stabilize mood and emotions. Menthol energizes emotions, so this is where Peppermint shines. The geraniol found in Geranium and Rose has clarifying properties for the emotions, while linalool both clarifies and calms, found in Coriander, Cilantro, Basil, Lavender, Petitgrain, Clary Sage, and Bergamot. More mood-stabilizing essential oils are those with santalol (Sandalwood), cedrol (Cedarwood), and patchoulol (Patchouli).

Aldehydes such as cinnamaldehyde, geranial, and neral calm the emotions and settle the mood while protecting the mind and body. Protective essential oils like Cinnamon and Cassia boast cinnamaldehyde, while soothing Melissa and Lemongrass primarily contain geranial and neral.

Ketones such as carvone, camphor, and menthone calm moods and promote mental concentration. Peppermint also has menthone in it, which energizes moods, while Dill and Spearmint have carvone, which also invigorates and energizes emotions.

Esters such as methyl salicylate, linalyl acetate, and neryl acetate aid in calming moods and restoring emotions while supporting hormones at the same time. Restoring essential oils like Wintergreen and Birch have methyl salicylate, while Helichrysum is composed primarily of neryl acetate. Lavender, Petitgrain, Clary Sage, and Bergamot calm the emotions with their primary constituent of linalyl acetate.

Emotional Triggers

Because our emotions are embedded in our physiological makeup, it makes sense that certain sights, smells, and experiences can trigger emotional releases. All these pent-up emotions can clog your emotional pathways, preventing you from feeling truly free. Essential oils allow your body and mind to release these pent-up emotions by stimulating your emotional brain via the limbic system. That is, you can *feel* the result of their aromas before you can mentally understand *why* you feel the way you do.

Every emotion, from anger to fear, anxiety to failure, grief to worthlessness, can be released by using the corresponding essential oil. A positive affirmation paired with an essential oil can be a powerful combination in releasing these pent-up emotions. Some of the favorite affirmations I use in my self-care rituals include:

- I am worthy.
- I am strong.
- I am confident.
- I love myself.
- I am beautiful.
- I am enough.

Whatever affirmation makes you feel more confident and powerful will help you reclaim control of your emotions and stabilize your mood. Try a combination of them, and record your results in your journal along with your emotional triggers.

How to Support Your Emotional Well-Being with Essential Oils

Because essential oils are so potent and powerful, inhaling them directly affects our limbic brain, which regulates emotional reactions. No wonder the aromas influence our emotions in such a profound way! Because the constituents of essential oils vary so widely, each oil is able to work in a unique way.

We often associate certain aromas with particular emotions, coloring our memories that get triggered only when the scent wafts our way again. Say, the aroma of cinnamon rolls baking in your grandmother's kitchen elicits feelings of warmth and comfort; the scent of wood smoke can cause fear and anxiety if you've been caught in a house fire. It is truly amazing how scents can transport us.

As mentioned, the three categories of essential oils that help stabilize mood are calming/soothing, energizing/uplifting, and grounding/balancing. Used individually, each is helpful in establishing a baseline for emotional balance, but used in combination, as recommended in the suggestions that follow or in the recipes, they bring the most success. Often, also, using the oils internally as well as aromatically provides the best support against emotional imbalance. Be persistent and consistent with their use, and experiment to find out which work for you in different situations.

Preferred Essential Oils

CALMING/SOOTHING

GERANIUM (*Pelargonium graveolens*)
- Calms the nerves and soothes the mind and body from excess stress
- Grounds emotions from worry, frustration, and stress

Aromatic Use
- Diffuse 3–4 drops.
- Add 1 drop to your palms, rub together, cup over nose, and inhale deeply. Rub the rest on your neck and shoulders or on face.

Topical Use
- Dilute 1–2 drops with a carrier oil and massage into the body.
- Apply after a shower.

YLANG YLANG (*Cananga odorata*)
- Calms the mind and body while uplifting your mood
- Boosts your mood to create a positive outlook on life
- Lessens feelings of tension and stress to allow for emotional balance

Aromatic Use
- Diffuse 3–4 drops.

Topical Use
- Dilute 1–2 drops with a carrier oil and apply to pulse points.
- Dilute 1–2 drops with a carrier oil and massage into tense areas of the body.

- Add 3–4 drops to ¼ cup Epsom salts and dissolve into a warm bath.

ROMAN CHAMOMILE (*Anthemis nobilis*)

- Enhances overall feelings of calm and relaxation for the mind and body
- Soothes the entire body while inspiring courage and self-esteem
- Comforts the mind and body when overwhelm begins to threaten imbalance

Aromatic Use

- Diffuse 3–4 drops.
- Inhale or diffuse while practicing deep-breathing techniques to reduce stress.

Topical Use

- Add 1–2 drops to your favorite moisturizer.
- Dilute 1–2 drops with a carrier oil and apply to your soles at bedtime.

Internal Use

- Add 1–2 drops to your favorite herbal tea.

LAVENDER (*Lavandula angustifolia*)

- Eases feelings of anxiety, tension, and stress by instilling an overall sense of calm
- Promotes total body relaxation and supports a restful night's sleep
- Allows your body to find peace amid the stress in your day

Aromatic Use

- Diffuse 3–4 drops.
- Add 1–2 drops to pillows and bedclothes before bedtime.
- Inhale directly from the bottle and practice deep breathing.

Topical Use

- Dilute 1–2 drops with a carrier oil and massage into any tense areas of the body.
- Add 3–4 drops to ½ cup Epsom salts and dissolve into a warm bath.

CLARY SAGE (*Salvia sclarea*)

- Relaxes and soothes the mind and body while calming emotions
- Reduces nervous tension and anxiety from emotional and hormonal imbalance
- Balances the body and mind to allow for relaxation

Aromatic Use

- Diffuse 2 drops with 2 drops of your favorite citrus oil.
- Diffuse 3–4 drops before bedtime.

Topical Use

- Dilute 1–2 drops with a carrier oil and massage into your abdomen.
- Dilute 1–2 drops with a carrier oil and massage into pulse points.
- Combine 2 drops Clary Sage, 2 drops Roman Chamomile, and 2 drops Lavender with ½ cup Epsom salts and dissolve into a warm bath.

MELISSA (*Melissa officinalis*)

- Alleviates anxiety, nervousness, and tension
- Uplifts and restores positive moods
- Calms and relaxes the mind and body

Aromatic Use

- Diffuse 3–4 drops at nighttime.
- Add 1 drop to your palms, rub together, cup over your nose, and inhale deeply.

Topical Use

- Dilute 1–2 drops with a carrier oil and massage into shoulders and neck.
- Dilute 1–2 drops with a carrier oil and massage into the temples and over pulse points.

COPAIBA (*Copaifera reticulata, C. officinalis, C. coriacea,* and *C. langsdorffii*)

- Soothes and calms anxiety and nervous tension
- Calms, soothes, and supports the nervous system while aiding in emotional balance
- Supports a variety of bodily systems to help your body to maintain balance

Aromatic Use

- Diffuse 3–4 drops.
- Inhale directly from the bottle.

Topical Use

- Dilute 1–2 drops with a carrier oil and massage into tense areas of the body.

JASMINE ABSOLUTE (*Jasminum grandiflorum*)

- Uplifts the emotions
- Enhances feelings of joy and peace while instilling self-confidence
- Promotes a positive outlook on life

Aromatic Use

- Diffuse 3–4 drops.

Topical Use

- Dilute 1–2 drops with a carrier oil and apply to pulse points.
- Dilute 1–2 drops with a carrier oil and massage into your soles in the morning.

BASIL (*Ocimum basilicum*)

- Alleviates nervous tension and anxiety in the mind and body
- Enhances mental focus and alertness while rejuvenating the mind and body
- Reduces muscle tension

Aromatic Use

- Diffuse 3–4 drops.
- Inhale directly from the bottle.

Topical Use
- Apply 1 diluted drop to fingertips and massage into temples.
- Dilute 1–2 drops with a carrier oil and massage into tense muscles. Add 1 drop of Wintergreen for a cooling and relaxing sensation.

ENERGIZING/UPLIFTING

BERGAMOT (*Citrus bergamia*)
- Calms and uplifts the mind and body while alleviating fatigue, tension, and anxiety
- Is perfect for massage blends and diffusing as well as internal calm when added to herbal tea

WILD ORANGE (*Citrus sinensis*)
- Energizing aroma that uplifts the mind and body while purifying the air
- Perfect addition to smoothies and water for internal support and detox

Aromatic Use
- Diffuse 2 drops Wild Orange with Peppermint and Frankincense, or other complementary essential oils.
- Breathe directly from the bottle.

Topical Use
- Add to massage blends or rollerball blends.

WARNING: Remember that citrus oils are phototoxic, so avoid direct sunlight for at least 12 hours with most citrus oils but up to 72 hours with Bergamot.

PEPPERMINT (*Mentha piperita*)
- Promotes energetic feelings by enlivening the senses
- Encourages healthy respiratory function to enhance your exercise routines
- Cools and invigorates skin that helps improve focus and alertness

Aromatic Use
- Diffuse 3–4 drops.
- Diffuse with Wild Orange for an energy boost.

Topical Use
- Add 1 drop each Peppermint, Wild Orange, and Frankincense to your palms, rub together, and inhale deeply.
- Dilute with a carrier oil and massage onto neck and shoulders.
- Dilute with a carrier oil and massage into fatigued and tense areas of the body.

GROUNDING/BALANCING

CEDARWOOD (*Juniperus virginiana*)
- Soothes and relaxes the mind and body to stabilize mood
- Instills confidence and promotes self-esteem
- Enhances feelings of overall wellness and vitality

Aromatic Use
- Diffuse 3–4 drops.
- Inhale directly from the bottle.

Topical Use
- Dilute 1–2 drops with a carrier oil and massage into chest.
- Dilute 1–2 drops with a carrier oil and massage into any tense areas of the body.

FRANKINCENSE (*Boswellia carterii, B. frereana*, and *B. sacra*)
- Supports overall peace and wellness for emotional balance
- Opens the mind and body for overall relaxation and grounding balance
- Aids in dissipating negativity and reducing stress while soothing and relaxing your emotions

Aromatic Use
- Diffuse 3–4 drops.
- Inhale directly from the bottle.

Topical Use
- Dilute 1–2 drops with a carrier oil and apply to your soles before bedtime.
- Dilute 1–2 drops with a carrier oil and massage into tense areas.

PATCHOULI (*Pogostemon cablin*)
- Stabilizes mood by grounding and balancing emotions
- Relieves feelings of tension and pent-up anger

Aromatic Use
- Diffuse 3–4 drops.
- Inhale directly from the bottle with deep breaths.

Topical Use
- Dilute 1–2 drops with a carrier oil, combine with Peppermint, and massage into the temples, behind the ears, and down the back of your neck.
- Dilute 1–2 drops with a carrier oil, combine with Vetiver, and massage into your soles before bedtime.

INDIAN SANDALWOOD (*Santalum album*)
- Enhances the mood by settling and stabilizing emotions
- Promotes grounding and uplifting, especially when used with meditation and prayer

Aromatic Use
- Diffuse 3–4 drops.
- Add 1 drop to the shower floor.

Topical Use
- Add 3–4 drops to ½ cup Epsom salts and dissolve into a warm bath.
- Dilute 1–2 drops with a carrier oil and massage into the back of your neck and your soles before bedtime.

VETIVER (*Vetiveria zizanioides*)
- Calms and grounds the mind and body to support emotional balance

- Zaps anxiety, nervousness, and intense moments of stress
- Promotes deep relaxation that calms emotions for a restful night's sleep

Aromatic Use

- Diffuse 2 drops Vetiver and 2 drops Lavender.
- Add 1 drop to palms, rub together, cup over nose, and inhale deeply. Massage the remainder into your neck and shoulder.

Topical Use

- Dilute 1–2 drops with a carrier oil and massage into your soles before bedtime.
- Add 3 drops to ¼ cup Epsom salts and dissolve in a warm bath.

Joanne's Story

Joanne, a forty-seven-year-old administrator for a non-profit organization and volunteer for her local food bank, came to me with concerns about occasional sadness and anxiousness. She was recently divorced after being married for twenty-two years, and although she kept herself busy, she was struggling to adjust to her new life. She felt isolated and sad most nights, was experiencing random panic attacks on her way home from work, had a hard time getting out of bed on the weekends, and began noticing hormonal changes. She wanted to address her low energy and fatigue.

Joanne was experiencing perimenopause and mild depression and anxiousness. **My recommendations were as follows:**

- Abundance and Gratitude Diffuser Blend (page 202) and gratitude journaling five days a week to provide a feeling of gratitude and happiness each morning.

- Schedule dates with friends, or attend social events throughout the weekend and in the evenings.
- Use essential oils throughout the day for support. Keep the Happy Bliss Inhaler Blend (page 203) or the Self-Love, Self-Care Diffuser Blend (page 203) out and schedule times to use them.
- Creating a morning ritual with essential oils. Start the day with the the Energize Your Mood Inhaler Blend (page 203) for energy and mood uplifting and continue to use it in the afternoon.
- Substitute coffee with matcha green tea. L-theanine reduces stress and feelings of anxiousness.
- Support gut health by incorporating whole foods for breakfast, lunch, and dinner.
- Exercise for 30 minutes three to four times a week to boost happy neurotransmitters and increase energy.
- Supplements: multivitamin, 2000 mg omega-3 fatty acids, 450 mg St. John's wort, 300 mg magnesium glycinate to support mood, hormone levels, and increase energy.
- Self-care rituals: Incorporate the Intense Deep-Breathing Ritual (page 205) during moments when anxious feelings arise.

Within six weeks, Joanne experienced less anxiety, fewer mood swings, and diminished depressed feelings, and she felt more balanced in her body. She also felt more content with her life and enjoyed spending time with her friends. She knew she was still adjusting to being single, but she really enjoyed her work and serving her community. The morning ritual and gratitude journaling were the perfect routine she had been missing, and the essential-oil blends helped her throughout the day and during times of need, particularly Lavender and Frankincense with sadness and emotional blends for energy and mood. "I had no idea that essential oils could help with my emotional moments, but they did! And they are so easy to use. I keep my favorite blends in my purse and pull them out at least four to five times a day. I love starting my morning with wild orange and bergamot. They really help me to get out of bed."

Essential Oil Blends

Aromatic Diffuser Blends

Positive Affirmation Diffuser Blend

3 drops Bergamot essential oil
2 drops Clary Sage essential oil
1 drop Wild Orange essential oil

Nix Anxious Feelings Diffuser Blend

2 drops Patchouli essential oil
2 drops Wild Orange essential oil
1 drop Ylang Ylang essential oil
1 drop Lavender essential oil

Abundance and Gratitude Diffuser Blend

2 drops Frankincense essential oil
2 drops Wild Orange essential oil
2 drops Peppermint essential oil

Emotional Release Diffuser Blend

2 drops Geranium essential oil
2 drops Bergamot essential oil

1 drop Lemongrass essential oil

1 drop Ylang Ylang essential oil

Self-Love, Self-Care Diffuser Blend

3 drops Bergamot essential oil

2 drops Cedarwood essential oil

1 drop Lavender essential oil

Aromatic Personal Inhaler Blends

Happy Bliss Inhaler Blend

7 drops Wild Orange essential oil

4 drops Grapefruit essential oil

4 drops Ylang Ylang essential oil

Energize Your Mood Inhaler Blend

5 drops Rosemary essential oil

5 drops Peppermint essential oil

5 drops Grapefruit essential oil

Calm and Ground Inhaler Blend

4 drops Lavender essential oil

4 drops Yarrow essential oil

4 drops Frankincense essential oil

3 drops Cedarwood essential oil

Topical Rollerball Blends

Overwhelm Reset Rollerball Blend

8 drops Geranium essential oil

8 drops Clary Sage essential oil

6 drops Cypress essential oil

3 drops Patchouli essential oil

3 drops Ylang Ylang essential oil

Carrier oil of choice

Add the essential oils to a 10 mL glass rollerball bottle and fill the rest with a carrier oil. Replace the rollerball top and cap, and then shake gently to blend. To use, apply to the back of the neck, temples, behind the ears, and on the wrists.

Emotional Balance Rollerball Blend

10 drops Geranium essential oil
5 drops Neroli essential oil
5 drops Jasmine essential oil
5 drops Ylang Ylang essential oil
Carrier oil of choice

Add essential oils to a 10 mL glass rollerball bottle and fill the rest with a carrier oil. Replace rollerball top and cap, and shake gently to blend. To use, apply to pulse points and inhale deeply.

Panic-Buster Rollerball Blend

8 drops Clary Sage essential oil
7 drops Lavender essential oil
5 drops Vetiver essential oil
5 drops Roman Chamomile essential oil
Carrier oil of choice

Add essential oils to a 10 mL glass rollerball bottle and fill the rest with a carrier oil. Replace rollerball top and cap, and shake gently to blend. To use, apply to pulse points and inhale deeply.

Self-Care Rituals for Emotional Balance

"Is This Serving Me?" Ritual

One of my all-time favorite questions is: "Is this serving me right now?" I love the concept of using a question to create a positive affirmation because it causes me to pause and examine the situation at hand. Sometimes, I find myself searching for a justification to keep doing what I'm doing, but more often than not, I am able to come to a screeching halt and dismiss something that isn't serving me. I give myself permission to just say no to whatever is causing me more harm than joy.

You can apply this question to just about every situation and even to concrete objects. If I put on a dress that for some reason I don't feel comfortable in, I ask, "Is this serving me?" Nope, it's not, because I'm going to spend all day with anxiety about how I feel and look in the outfit. If I don't love it and it doesn't make me feel confident, then it's time to purge!

What about that glass of wine after a rough day? Is it serving me? When I consider that I haven't eaten dinner, have spent the day surviving on sugar-laden snacks, and have reached levels of stress that I've dealt with for hours, no . . . this glass of wine will do nothing when I could have a calming mug of herbal tea and healthy dinner instead. Trigger avoided.

Once you see this question as a ritual, it will become second nature to ask it whenever the need arises. I've found it to be an incredibly useful tool for decision-making.

Intense Deep-Breathing Ritual

You have already learned my favorite deep-breathing technique (see Chapter 5). I turn to it whenever I feel a bad mood or any feeling of being overwhelmed. In fact, I recommend making this a daily ritual, multiple times a day, and as much as you need during times of intense stress. Let the rhythm of your breaths complement the rush of air being sucked in through your nostrils, billowing into the deep recesses of your lungs, and being slowly let out through your mouth. Hang in the pauses between the inhales and the exhales, and try to work up to counting to ten in those moments of calm.

As you get even better at this ritual, you can use those pauses to meditate and focus on positive affirmations or to offer a quick prayer of thanks and gratitude. Adding high-quality essential oils to your breathing will give you a combination that rejuvenates both mind and body while supporting a positive mood and a restored confidence.

Banish Feeling Overwhelmed Ritual

Not long ago, I had a five-minute meltdown when I found myself smacked in the face with feelings of being utterly overwhelmed. Luckily, I reached for my essential-oil kit to pull out my Overwhelm Reset Rollerball Blend (page 203). With shaking hands, I uncapped the bottle and deeply inhaled while closing my eyes and practicing the Intense Deep-Breathing Ritual. I rolled some into the palms of my hand, cupped it over my nose, and began to calm myself enough to hang in the pauses. I focused on gratitude and my blessings as my emotions began to stabilize. When I opened my eyes, I rolled more onto my pulse points and took a moment to continue breathing and being in the moment. That panic attack had really scared me. But thankfully I had the tools to find my center again.

I encourage you to prepare yourself for moments like this. Find the essential oils that support you best and have them ready and in an essential-oil kit for on-the-go needs.

Preserving-the-Peace Partner Ritual

Even though I teach a life-transforming plan, life still gets the best of me every now and then. It's then that I have a moment, or make an adjustment, or just need some time to stop and breathe. Luckily, I'm blessed to have a husband who sees my triggers, recognizes my body's cries for help sometimes before I do, and knows when to support me. He hands me my favorite rollerball blend and tells me everything is going to be okay. He diffuses the anxiety for me, he massages me to eliminate the kinks, and he keeps me balanced when I ignore my triggers. And I do the same for him. It's an "oily" partnership in peace, so we can continue to carry on the life we love and keep each other healthy in the process.

Find your someone and make him or her a partner in preserving the peace. It can be a friend, a spiritual leader, a partner, a spouse—anyone who can check in with you, recognize your needs, and know the questions to ask or essential oils to hand you when anxiety threatens to spin you into a whirlwind. You can do the same for him or her. Set a regular time to check in with one another and talk about how you are doing—and what oils you are using!

CHAPTER 12

Cognitive Issues: Memory and Concentration

P ray, love, remember," says Ophelia in Shakespeare's *Hamlet*, as she references rosemary as an herb of remembrance. She wasn't wrong—one of the simplest ways to increase memory, concentration, and focus is to open a bottle of Rosemary essential oil and breathe it in deeply. But Shakespeare couldn't have proven what researchers recently have—that Rosemary essential oil is able to immediately influence memory, up to 75 percent more simply by inhaling it, owing to its primary constituent, 1,8-cineole. More studies have since shown its ability to enhance long-term memory and increase alertness. Even better is the discovery that inhaling the aroma of Rosemary essential oil is enough to transport 1,8-cineole into the bloodstream—through the olfactory system. As a result, it can directly affect the neurotransmitter acetylcholine (ACh) that neurons use to send messages to one another, influencing memory, cognition, and learning.

Degenerative brain disorders are a scary prospect as we age—

especially if they appear in our family lineage. According to a study reported in the journal *Neuropharmacology* in March 2016, linalool, a primary constituent of essential oils like Basil, Cilantro, Clary Sage, Coriander, and Lavender, when taken internally, helps to improve learning, memory, and overall cognitive functioning when used over time. When you combine internal use of essential oils with diffusion or aromatic use, the powerful effect that it can have on the mind and body shows great potential for the future.

But when you're standing in the middle of your living room unable to figure out why you just found your keys in the dishwasher, it's scary. When you call your kids by the wrong name or can't remember the word for "dryer," it's embarrassing. My patients come to me in a hot panic, convinced that they are descending into dementia. Luckily, I'm usually able to reassure them that we will get to the root of the problem and that dementia is hardly likely.

Obviously, the mind-body connection is paramount in supporting an overall sense of wellness and vitality, but there are environmental and internal conditions that can greatly affect our ability to focus. Some of them may be surprising and others will make sense based on what you've already learned in this book. Even if you haven't had any symptoms of decreased focus or memory yet, you can still employ the techniques in this chapter to prevent what may be coming in your future.

The Why Behind Cognitive Issues

Stress

Stress particularly affects the neurotransmitter acetylcholine, reducing its ability to aid in memory formation. When this neurotransmitter is impaired, we can also experience increased anxiety, inflammation, disrupted sleep patterns, digestive issues, and pancreatic hormone function. We might also be at an increased risk for brain-related diseases such as Parkinson's disease and Alzheimer's disease.

Emotional Health

As you have just read, acetylcholine is required for memory formation, but it can take days to return to normal levels when affected by traumatic events, whether physical or emotional. This is why a traumatic event can leave your mind in limbo for a while as you try to process what happened. This makes sense when you consider how acute stress events can potentially cause depression, amnesia, or other memory-related issues.

Aging

Aging tends to reduce the ability to process information and reason, as well as affecting a variety of memory-related functions. On the other hand, the wisdom we acquire based on experience does benefit us in the long run. In addition, the sense of smell tends to decrease with age, making researchers wonder if cognitive impairment may be related to olfactory decline. Luckily, you can use essential oils to activate all the brain areas involved in memory processing.

Diet

It goes without saying that not properly fueling your body with the macro- and micronutrients you need will dramatically influence your brain power. In addition, not hydrating well throughout the day can affect mental focus. Stick to the dietary recommendations in this book, especially in the 14-Day Rescue Plan, and I promise you will see an improvement in your brain power.

Gut Health

You will see in the next chapter how the gut influences cognition. Known as the "second brain," the gut is always sending messages to the brain to keep the body healthy and balanced. Imbalanced gut flora affect the production of neurotransmitters like serotonin, which influence mood, and food sensitivities to gluten or dairy, or imbalances in the gut caused by candida or other issues, can affect how you think.

Sleep

Brain growth and neuroplasticity rely on appropriate amounts of sleep to keep your cognitive powers sharp. Synaptic connections are also strengthened during restful sleep, so do whatever you can to support your body's circadian rhythms and get the proper amount of sleep every night. For more on this, refer to Chapter 7.

Your Hormones for Cognitive Issues

Cortisol and Chronic Stress

Hello again, high cortisol levels! Increased cortisol may enhance the ability to consolidate short-term memory, but it has the opposite effect on accessing, contextualizing, storing, and retrieving long-term memories. When high levels of cortisol contribute to anxiety and depression, synapses are lost in the prefrontal cortex, the area that houses short-term memory, thus allowing for communication throughout the brain. Synapses process, store, and recall information, but prolonged stress combined with age can make them shrink and disappear—what's called a "weathering of the brain." As a result, your brain has to work harder to create and sustain memories, and even harder to retrieve them.

Thyroid Issues

Both hyperthyroidism and hypothyroidism can affect the ability to concentrate and to form and retain memories. This is often referred to as "brain fog." Don't overlook those symptoms if you haven't had your thyroid levels tested.

Estrogen and Progesterone

Normal hormone function allows estrogen to help regulate cortisol levels, which in turn support healthy neurotransmitter functioning; this means estrogen helps you effectively make decisions while supporting short-term memory. (Many estrogen receptors are found in the hippocampus, and the prefrontal cortex contains many estrogen receptors, where episodic and working memory take place.) Likewise, progesterone protects the brain by allowing increased blood flow to support mental function. It also helps keep free radical damage at bay.

When these hormone levels drop with age, memory loss and cognitive impairment naturally result; less estrogen means less ability to regulate cortisol. This causes problems with short-term recall and verbal tasks.

Emotional Triggers for Cognitive Issues

The simplest way to explain how emotions affect your memory appears in what I call "clouding." When significant emotional events occur close to or simultaneously with other events and/or information, the emotions cloud the details, causing an altered state of remembrance. For women, the effect is even stronger. After 9/11, for example, many people found that certain precise details of the disaster were fixed in their minds, while they had no memory of how they got home that evening or what they did in the days following that awful event. Your current mood also affects your ability to remember details, so a pleasant mood will more often tone the memory as pleasant as well. The stronger the emotions, the more likely you are to remember specific details about an event. Obviously, this means that mental disorders such as depression or anxiety will also cloud your memories.

When intensely stressful or fearful experiences take place, our bodies respond by releasing cortisol to help us handle the situation. In the same instance, however, oxytocin is also released, thereby intensifying the memory. The two hormones work together in the formation of deep-seated, emotionally traumatic long-term memories that may help us to avoid a similar situation in the future. Whenever the memory is triggered, however, cortisol levels also spike, causing the body to almost "relive" the moment and experience the same stressful emotions. This is the basis for anxiety, panic attacks, and post-traumatic stress disorder (PTSD).

How to Support Your Cognitive Issues with Essential Oils

Preferred Essential Oils

ROSEMARY (*Rosmarinus officinalis*)
- Increases alertness and focus, aiding in memory and concentration
- Stimulates the mind and body to help with cognitive performance
- Enhances the mood to allow for proper brain function

Aromatic Use
- Diffuse 3–4 drops to enhance mental focus and maintain concentration.
- Inhale directly from the bottle for an instantaneous brain boost.

Topical Use
- Dilute 1–2 drops with a carrier oil and massage into the body to reduce tension while rejuvenating the mind and body. Mix with Lavender for a de-stressing experience.
- Add 2 drops Rosemary and 2 drops Frankincense to ¼ cup Epsom salts and swirl into a warm bath to dissolve.

BASIL (*Ocimum basilicum*)

- Encourages mental alertness and focus while alleviating anxiety
- Relieves tension and stress while restoring relief and calm
- Alleviates distracting symptoms from your menstrual cycle

Aromatic Use

- Diffuse 3–4 drops.
- Inhale directly from the bottle.

Topical Use

- Dilute 1–2 drops with a carrier oil and massage into tense areas of the body, especially the temples and the neck. Add 1 drop Wintergreen for an even deeper effect.
- Dilute 1–2 drops with a carrier oil and massage into the abdomen during your menstrual cycle.

Citrus Essential Oils

The uses of these citrus essential oils are all similar and appear with the Wild Orange listing.

BERGAMOT (*Citrus bergamia*)

- Calms and uplifts the mind and body while alleviating fatigue, tension, and anxiety
- Perfect for massage blends and diffusing as well as internal calm when added to black herbal tea

LEMON (*Citrus limon*)

- Promotes a positive mood while invigorating the mind and body
- Perfect addition to smoothies and water for internal support, detox, and digestion

LIME (*Citrus aurantifolia*)

- Stimulates the mind and body while uplifting mood and refreshing the senses

- Promotes emotional health and well-being
- Perfect addition to smoothies and water for internal support and detox

WILD ORANGE (*Citrus sinensis*)

- Energizing aroma that uplifts the mind and body while purifying the air
- Perfect addition to smoothies and water for internal support and detox

Aromatic Use
- Diffuse 2 drops citrus oil with Peppermint and Frankincense, or other complementary essential oils.
- Inhale directly from the bottle.

Topical Use
- Add to massage blends or rollerball blends.

WARNING: Remember that citrus oils are phototoxic, so avoid direct sunlight for at least 12 hours with most citrus oils but up to 72 hours with Bergamot.

JUNIPER BERRY (*Juniperus communis*)

- Supports healthy internal organ function, especially for the kidneys and urinary tract
- Grounds and calms the mind and body
- Alleviates feelings of overwhelm to aid the mind in focusing

Aromatic Use
- Diffuse 3–4 drops. Pair with Bergamot to uplift the emotions and create a positive atmosphere.

Topical Use
- Dilute 1–2 drops with a carrier oil and massage into tense areas of the body.
- Dilute 1–2 drops with a carrier oil and add to your palms, rub together, cup over your nose, and deeply inhale. Rub the remainder on your neck and shoulders.

MELISSA (*Melissa officinalis*)

- Increases alertness while improving accuracy and attention
- Calms the mind and body and reduces tension, especially those with anxiety and insomnia
- Supports a healthy immune system when taken internally

Aromatic Use

- Diffuse 3–4 drops to alleviate feelings of tension and nervousness in the body.
- Diffuse at night with Lavender to support a relaxing and restful night's sleep that supports your emotions.
- Inhale directly from the body to find calm during moments of anxiety.

Topical Use

- Dilute 1–2 drops with a carrier oil and massage into the forehead, shoulders, and chest.
- Add a drop to your favorite moisturizer and massage into face and body.

LAVENDER (*Lavandula angustifolia*)

- Reduces stress, which helps the mind calm for focus on tasks
- Balances the emotions and calms the mind to allow for focus and mood support
- Supports a restful night's sleep to nourish and support brain function

Aromatic Use

- Diffuse 3–4 drops at night.
- Inhale directly from the bottle.
- Add a drop or two to bedclothes before bedtime.

Topical Use

- Dilute 1–2 drops with a carrier oil and massage into tense areas.
- Add 3–4 drops to ½ cup Epsom salts and swirl into a warm bath.

FRANKINCENSE (*Boswellia carterii, B. frereana, and B. sacra*)

- Supports healthy cellular function in the body, especially the central nervous system
- Provides feelings of peace and relaxation to promote overall vitality
- Sustains feelings of positivity and focus to keep you balanced and focused throughout the day

Aromatic Use

- Diffuse 3–4 drops.
- Diffuse during yoga or exercise.

Topical Use

- Dilute 1–2 drops with a carrier oil and apply to your soles.
- Dilute 1–2 drops with a carrier oil and massage where needed.

VETIVER (*Vetiveria zizanioides*)

- Calms and grounds intense emotions while sustaining vitality
- Supports a healthy immune system
- Enhances mental performance and focus to support concentration

Aromatic Use

- Diffuse 3–4 drops.

Topical Use

- Dilute 1–2 drops with a carrier oil and massage into tense areas.
- Dilute 1–2 drops with a carrier oil and apply to your soles after a stressful experience and before bedtime.
- Add 3 drops to ¼ cup Epsom salts and dissolve into a warm bath.

PEPPERMINT (*Mentha piperita*)

- Stimulates mental focus and energy by enlivening the senses
- Encourages healthy respiratory function to enhance your deep breathing rituals

- Cools and invigorates skin that helps improve focus, concentration, and mental performance

Aromatic Use
- Diffuse 3–4 drops.
- Diffuse with Wild Orange for an energy boost.

Topical Use
- Add 1 drop each of Peppermint, Wild Orange, and Frankincense to your palms, rub together, and inhale deeply.
- Dilute 1–2 drops with a carrier oil and massage onto neck and shoulders.
- Dilute 1–2 drops with a carrier oil and massage into fatigued and tense areas of the body.

Patricia's Story

Patricia was fifty-two years old when she came to me, concerned with recent trouble concentrating and staying motivated at work. Patricia was a human resources analyst, working at a computer all day crunching numbers; she was worried that her occasional forgetfulness was affecting her performance, and that co-workers would notice. She began relying on coffee and protein bars in the middle of the day to keep her focused and motivated, but that didn't always work. She felt her new afternoon habits were actually affecting her energy levels later in the evening, and her goal was to feel more focused, energized, and less stressed.

Patricia presented with brain fog, low fluctuating estrogen levels due to menopause, and increased cortisol levels in the evening. **My recommendations were as follows:**

- For afternoon energy slumps and cravings, inhale the Crave-Control Rollerball Blend (page 147) every hour during a 5-minute stretch break.
- For stress at work, apply the Motivation Rollerball Blend (page 222) on the wrist and palms and take 3 to 5 deep belly breaths.

For more restful sleep, diffuse the

- Deep Relaxation Diffuser Blend (page 127) 2 hours before bed. Apply Lavender and Clary Sage to her neck and feet before going to bed.
- Start each morning with a 5-minute meditation and Focus and Alert Diffuser Blend (page 220) to help with stress and provide mental clarity at the start of the day.
- Use the Morning Boost Inhaler Blend (page 106) at work to provide instant focus and energy.
- Cardiovascular and strength training exercise two to three times a week for 30 minutes and walking and/or yoga one to two times a week to increase endorphins, get more glucose and oxygen flowing to the brain, and burn off excess cortisol.
- Increase water intake by carrying a large water bottle and refilling it often at work.
- Substitute matcha for coffee and cut out snacking in the afternoon. The L-theanine in green tea reduces stress without causing sedation.
- Follow the 14-Day Rescue Plan to remove any foods that could cause brain fog and increase brain-boosting whole foods.
- Supplements: a multivitamin, 500 mg of rhodiola, 2000 mg of omega-3 fatty acid to lower stress

levels and support brain function, and 1500 mg maca added to a morning green smoothie.

Within four weeks, Patricia experienced significantly less brain fog and stress at work. She was falling asleep easier at night, as she did not come home anxious about her workday. She lost seven pounds and experienced more energy, especially after taking five-minute breaks throughout her workday with the Focus and Alert Diffuser Blend (see below). Her mid-afternoon caffeine cravings were gone and her memory felt restored. When I asked how she felt overall, she replied, "I had no idea that essential oils could help to improve mood, memory, and energy levels. I feel significantly more productive at work and the brain fog cloud has lifted. I am going to continue to take essential oil breaks every hour. That one habit has made all the difference."

Essential Oil Blends

Aromatic Diffuser Blends

Memory-Boosting Diffuser Blend

4 drops Juniper Berry essential oil
3 drops Rosemary essential oil
3 drops Bergamot essential oil

Anytime Energizer Boost Diffuser Blend

3 drops Peppermint essential oil
3 drops Wild Orange essential oil

Focus and Alert Diffuser Blend

2 drops Frankincense essential oil
2 drops Peppermint essential oil
2 drops Rosemary essential oil

Focus and Memory Diffuser Blend

3 drops Rosemary essential oil

2 drops Spearmint essential oil

2 drops Lemon essential oil

1 drop Ylang Ylang essential oil

Aromatic Personal Inhaler Blends

Mental Focus Inhaler Blend

8 drops Wild Orange essential oil

7 drops Peppermint essential oil

Ultimate Focus Inhaler Blend

6 drops Lemon or Grapefruit essential oil

3 drops Basil essential oil

3 drops Rosemary essential oil

2 drops Frankincense essential oil

Aromatic Room Spray

Uplifting Focus Room Spray

3 drops Vetiver essential oil

3 drops Rosemary essential oil

3 drops Lemon or Bergamot essential oil

3 drops Peppermint essential oil

2 tablespoons witch hazel

2 tablespoons distilled water

Add essential oils to a 2-ounce glass spray bottle and fill the rest of the way with water and witch hazel. Replace spray top and shake to blend. To use, shake and spritz in the air, on your clothes, or around the room.

Topical Rollerball Blends

Focus and Concentrate Rollerball Blend

10 drops Lavender essential oil

8 drops Grapefruit essential oil

3 drops Basil essential oil

3 drops Peppermint essential oil

Carrier oil of choice

Add the essential oils to a 10 mL glass rollerball bottle and fill the rest with a carrier oil. Replace the rollerball top and cap, and shake gently to blend. To use, apply to temples and massage in gently at least twice a day.

Motivation Rollerball Blend

5 drops Basil essential oil

10 drops Grapefruit essential oil

10 drops Wild Orange essential oil

In a 10 mL glass rollerball bottle, add the essential oils and fill the rest of the way with a carrier oil. Replace the rollerball top and cap, and then shake gently to combine. To use, roll on the palms, wrists, and ankles.

Confidence and Creativity Rollerball Blend

8 drops Bergamot essential oil

6 drops Spearmint essential oil

4 drops Clary Sage essential oil

4 drops Melissa or Geranium essential oil

Carrier oil of choice

Add the essential oils to a 10 mL glass rollerball bottle and fill the rest of the way with a carrier oil. Replace the rollerball top and cap, and shake gently to blend. To use, roll behind the ears, down neck, and on wrists.

Supplements That Support Cognition

Curcumin is found in turmeric, a popular Indian spice used in both Eastern medicine and Ayurveda. Curcumin's ability to increase blood flow to the brain and body reduces inflammation, which may be why it has shown promise in the treatment and prevention of a number of inflammatory brain-related disorders such as Alzheimer's and dementia—amazingly showing results in some studies in under an hour's time. It also helps to boost memory, balance mood disorders, and lower stress levels. As a spice, you can use it in your cooking, but it needs to be linked with a healthy fat. Choose high-quality, organic curcumin free of additives and fillers.

Matcha Green Tea has been used for thousands of years in Chinese healing and offers incredible support on many different levels. More potent than regular green tea, matcha delivers 100 percent of its nutrients and benefits because it's made from the entire tea leaf. With ten times more antioxidants than green tea, matcha helps to rid the body of free radicals that attack at a cellular level. One cup of matcha tea provides L-theanine, an amino acid that boosts mental clarity, as well as epigallocatechin gallate (EGCG), a polyphenol that works synergistically with L-theanine to support and increase brain health.

Rhodiola Rosea is an adaptogenic herb that can help to fight the body's stressors and revitalize overall wellness. It helps to increase focus, fight fatigue, and enhance your mood.

Vitamin B$_{12}$ is an essential vitamin necessary for energy production and many other supportive tasks, such as immune function, blood formation, DNA synthesis, and digestion. Deficiencies leave you feeling weak and easily fatigued, contributing to symptoms like muscle weakness, lack of focus and concentration, mood issues, and lack of motivation.

Vitamin D, which people commonly are deficient in, can easily be obtained with fifteen to twenty minutes of direct sun exposure each day, as well as through diet and supplementation. Vitamin D helps brain health by supporting the creation of new neural pathways, and also increases natural levels of dopamine and serotonin, which are essential for keeping your mood balanced and favorable; without them, you may be left depressed and fatigued. More drastic deficiency in this vitamin can contribute to severe health issues, such as cancer, depression, or hypothyroidism.

Omega-3 Fatty Acids (DHA and EPA) are vital for the maintenance of normal brain function throughout life. They are abundant in the fatty cell membranes of brain cells, preserving cell membrane health, reducing inflammation and facilitating communication between nerve cells. Most people don't need a supplement if they eat two or more servings of a fatty fish per week. If not, a supplement will help reduce inflammation and improve neural communication. DHA has proven to increase brain function, while EPA decreases inflammation to allow for increased blood flow. It has even been found to be successful in helping those recovering from traumatic brain injuries.

Bacopa Monnieri has been used for thousands of years in Ayurvedic practices. It aids in cognition and memory function, and it decreases inflammation in the brain. In order to have success, however, you need to take this supplement for at least four to six weeks before you will see any real results.

Self-Care Rituals for Cognitive Issues

Even though inhaling Rosemary essential oil can drastically improve your memory by at least 75 percent, there is no one easy fix for supporting overall cognitive function. Instead, as with everything else, ensure that your brain gets what it needs with your attention to proper nutrition, sleep, stress management, and a lower toxic load. Because stress greatly affects your ability to focus and concentrate, be sure to incorporate some of the self-care rituals from Chapter 5 as well as these rituals for keeping your mind sharp.

Go Outside Ritual

Being surrounded by nature and breathing in fresh air can wake up your brain right away. I love to go outside when I'm feeling sluggish, as this not only improves my energy levels but also helps clear my head, improves my mood, and gives me the vitamin D I need. If you can't get outside, try finding a location that stabilizes or enhances your mood. Being stuck in a place that doesn't bring you joy will cloud your memory and interfere with focus. I recommend diffusing your favorite focus-enhancing essential oil blend to make you feel better.

Think of Your Brain as a Muscle Ritual

Scientists used to believe that the neurons, or brain cells, you had were finite, but your brain is remarkably adaptable and new neural connections are always forming. One of the best ways to charge up your brain power is with specific exercises that trigger intense brain activity while also working your muscles. A great way to do this is with an activity, such as dance or any kind of workout with constantly changing routines, forcing your mind to count and think as you move. Or, try doing moves at home with your eyes closed—it's really not easy at first! Varying your exercise routines will not only stimulate your brain but also keep you from getting bored.

Exercise Your Mind Ritual

I have lots of friends who love to do crossword puzzles, number games like Sudoku, or brain teasers. It's very satisfying to solve a puzzle, and it's just as satisfying to know that memory games like these, even if done for just a few minutes every day, are an excellent way to fire up your brain. You can also get apps to game shows like *Jeopardy!* so you can test your memory skills. Inhaling Rosemary or Peppermint before you start your game, or diffusing your favorite brain-boosting blend, can help you to focus and solve the puzzle in record time. Lastly, consider meditation five to ten minutes a day to strengthen your brain power and reduce stress.

CHAPTER 13

Digestive Issues

Almost every woman I've treated over the years has come to me with individual issues, but just about every one mentions one topic in particular: digestive distress. As was discussed in Chapter 5, stress causes the digestive system to shut down in favor of survival, so it's no surprise that this is a common complaint.

Being stressed and overworked manifests as stomachaches and digestive distress, most often described as either "knots in my stomach" or "looseness." For me, it's one of the first signs that my body is getting off-track. A sluggish digestive system has always been my curse since I was a little girl, and I am cognizant of the importance of diet and exercise for healthy digestion. Also, I watch that my stress levels don't get so elevated that they trigger the release of too much cortisol. Once that happens, it's hard to recover, let alone its becoming a symptom of other problems, such as toxic load (which is discussed in Chapter 14), diet issues, or even an oncoming illness owing to a weakened immune system.

Thankfully, one deep breath from a bottle of Peppermint oil eases nausea, opens respiratory pathways, and awakens the senses. One drop of Peppermint massaged into the abdomen relaxes tense digestive muscles and releases the knots in the stomach contributing to loose stools or constipation, while simultaneously supplying a beneficial aromatic experience. Two drops of Peppermint taken internally in a veggie capsule alleviates severe digestive distress and promotes healthy functioning of the whole system. And that's just *one* essential oil. Wait until you see the power and potency of some of the digestive blends in this chapter!

The Why *Behind Digestive Issues*

Many of us are living with chronic digestive issues that we consider normal. When the digestive system isn't functioning properly, though, you can suffer from bloating, irritable bowel syndrome, constipation, and other digestive issues, as well as cardiovascular disease and osteoporosis. Doctors are often quick to prescribe medications that may alleviate some symptoms, or suggest a diet that only targets one problem. Again, this is a situation where the root cause must be uncovered and addressed for your digestive issues to improve or disappear.

Your Second Brain

Most of us assume that all knowledge and know-how to power our bodies originates in our brains, but there is another system at play: our digestive system. The enteric nervous system contains over 100 million neurons that enable us to "feel" a variety of functions happening on a daily basis. Even more interesting is that this "second brain" can function independently, owing to its ability to carry out its digestive functions while also sending messages to the brain. So, all of those "gut feelings" you've had may not have been so trivial after all. Trusting your gut may be the smartest thing you can do.

Often, we assume that our brains cause our gut to overact, but actually the opposite is true. For every one message that the brain sends to the gut, nine messages leave the gut for the brain. Everything from fullness and satiety to nausea and digestive upset are triggered in the gut and sent to the brain as danger messages. Even more interesting is that even when the brain doesn't respond in enough time to these messages, the enteric nervous system can take over and manage the issues in the gut.

Containing more than thirty neurotransmitters, the gut influences our emotional makeup more than we realize. In fact, your gut produces 95 percent of your serotonin, which functions much like a neurotransmitter and keeps your moods and digestive system running smoothly. When there is an imbalance, however, this can cause problems like irritable bowel syndrome or depression. With most of your immune system focused on the gut in order to flush out bad bacteria and foreign invaders, it's no wonder that the second brain plays such a large role in physiological functioning.

The Other Gut Influencers

The first step in reclaiming your gut health is to get your stress levels under control, as was described in Chapter 5. But there are other considerations to be aware of as well.

Antibacterial Cleansers. The antimicrobial agent triclosan was finally banned from use in hand sanitizers and cleaning products in 2016, but it was used for enough years to wipe out good bacteria as well as bad, and generally increased people's antibiotic resistance. Just use soap and water, reserving antibacterial solutions for emergency situations when you aren't able to suds up.

Diet. You are what you eat; what you fuel your body with directly affects your gut microbiome. When you focus on an organic, plant-based, whole foods and high-fiber diet with grass-fed animal protein, you help keep your gut functioning by supporting this microbiome and enabling proper nutrient absorption. Cutting out processed foods, sugars, caffeine, and even dairy and gluten can help your gut to reclaim control. Pairing a healthy protein with a complex carbohydrate every time you eat allows you to stay fuller longer and get the fiber you need.

In addition, research has shown that increasing tryptophan levels in your diet will support serotonin production. The highest levels of tryptophan are found not in turkey but in seaweed (like spirulina), spinach, seeds and nuts (chia, sunflower, flax, pistachio), crustaceans (lobster, shrimp, and crab), wild game (elk, rabbit, lean beef, goat, wild boar), chicken (and turkey), fish (halibut, tuna), eggs, and beans/lentils.

Antibiotic medications. Bacteria are constantly evolving, so overuse of antibiotics allows them, over time, to become resistant and render these medications useless—which is why overprescription of antibiotics is a global crisis. It is so dire that the federal government issued a National Action Plan to Combat Antibiotic-Resistant Bacteria. It is absolutely shocking that the prescription of one in three antibiotics is medically unnecessary. The problem is created both by patients who demand a quick fix when an illness is viral (and will never respond to antibiotics) and by doctors too willing to prescribe antibiotics "just in case." Factor in the antibiotics we consume as a by-product of the meat and poultry we eat, and an overabundance can easily overwhelm your body.

Antibiotics are designed to kill the bacteria in our guts, both harmful and healthy, in order to fight off the bad bugs. When we don't repopulate the over 100 *trillion* beneficial bacteria inside of our guts, our microbiome suffers. This also sets up the perfect growing conditions for unhealthy bacteria, such as *Candida albicans*, or yeast that can eventually affect the entire body; if serotonin levels are low, we are left battling yeast overgrowth on our own. Note that antibiotics aren't the only medication to be concerned about. Most medications have negative consequences on our microbiome as well.

Prebiotics and Probiotics. While many of us have heard of probiotics, *prebiotics* may be a new term. Prebiotic fiber has the ability to nourish the healthy bacteria in our microbiome and keep them thriving. Probiotics help to replenish the destruction of good bacteria. Adding a variety of fermented foods that contain probiotics can make a profound difference in your gut health. Look for fermented foods like kefir, sauerkraut, kombucha, and kimchi. Taking a probiotic supplement might be an easier option, but do your research and choose one with several different viable strains.

Sleep. Most digestion takes place while you're sleeping, so getting a restful night's sleep will allow your body to complete all of its daily cellular processes.

Self-Care Rituals. Nurturing your mind and body with self-care rituals will enable your body to de-stress and will greatly help improve your digestive issues.

Your Hormones for Digestive Issues

The Cortisol–Stress Connection

As you know, cortisol is the main hormone associated with stress. Excess levels for prolonged periods of time can cause the digestive system to shut down in favor of dealing with the particular stressor at hand. Your body will always favor survival over digestive function. This can disrupt the brain–gut axis and cause a number of digestive difficulties, such as inflammatory bowel disease (IBD), irritable bowel syndrome (IBS), gastroesophageal reflux disease (GERD), ulcers, and other issues. In addition, stress can activate corticotropin-releasing factor (CRF) responsible for regulating both upper and lower gastrointestinal tracts. As the primary neuro-hormone affecting the HPA axis, it has a huge effect on how the gut responds to stress.

Entrenched stress directly aggravates the trillions of healthy gut bacteria. It also weakens the lining of the gut, leaving it susceptible to leaky gut, nutritional deficiencies, autoimmune disease, and more.

The Serotonin–Gut Connection

Since nearly all your serotonin is produced in your gut, imbalanced levels will affect your mood, sleep, libido (excess levels decrease sexual desire), and overall health. If those levels are low or altered, serotonin can also trigger depression. If you have been prescribed antidepressants, many of these drugs inhibit the uptake of serotonin in both the enteric nervous system and the central nervous system. This causes a misdirection of serotonin to a localized area of nerve cells that eventually become desensitized to the onslaught, and your digestive system effectively gets stuck. It is no surprise that a huge complaint from those beginning antidepressants is nausea and diarrhea, followed by constipation. Interestingly, it has been found that those who don't have those symptoms aren't taking their medication correctly.

The Insulin–Digestive Connection

Produced by the pancreas, insulin allows the mitochondria to convert glucose into usable energy. When you eat, carbohydrates are converted to glucose and sent into the bloodstream, causing blood sugar levels to increase; in turn, this triggers the pancreas to produce insulin in order to direct the glucose where needed. A balanced diet containing appropriate levels of carbs enables insulin to properly function, keeping the blood sugar levels in balance and allowing enough glucose for cellular energy, as well as for storage for future needs. (This storage takes place in the liver, muscles, and fat cells as glycogen, which is used as fuel between meals.) The feedback loop between insulin and glycogen keeps blood sugar levels balanced and ensures that your body has a steady stream of energy.

Exocrine cells produced by the pancreas allow digestive enzymes to be released through ducts directly into the small intestine. These enzymes break down foods into nutrients so that the smaller nutrient molecules can be effectively absorbed into the bloodstream via the intestinal walls. The pancreatic enzymes rely on many other enzymes in order to properly digest food. The problem occurs when pancreatic hormones aren't able to do their job of balancing blood sugar, often because of improper diet, overeating, obesity, sugar addiction, and heavy use of alcohol. In addition, chronic stress detrimentally affects pancreatic function.

In Type 1 diabetes, which is genetic, the pancreas stops producing insulin, so daily doses must be given or the patient will die. In Type 2 diabetes, which can also be genetic but is usually caused by lifestyle factors (such as obesity and/or lack of physical activity), the body's cells no longer recognize insulin, and erratic blood sugar levels cause serious and sometimes lasting damage. Diabetes directly relates to cardiovascular disease, kidney failure, eye damage, blood vessel damage, neuropathy, and other serious health issues.

This is why it's so important to pay attention to how and what you eat. Increased blood sugar levels can cause constipation or diarrhea, as well as nausea and digestive distress—and an inability to properly absorb the nutrients we need. You would think this means weight loss, but the opposite is true. Excess belly fat and obesity often develop because the body cannot rid itself of excess amounts of sugar, inhibiting proper cellular function. This causes compromised circulatory and immune issues, making you more susceptible to illness.

Emotional Triggers for Digestive Issues

Thanks to the brain–gut connection, it should be no surprise that emotional triggers affect your digestion. When we begin to pay more attention to our gut instead of becoming irritated and more stressed about symptoms, we can begin to get to the root cause of our digestive issues. Rather than being physical in nature, digestive problems may truly be emotional in origin. We all know the clenched feeling we get deep in our bellies whenever stress kicks in or anxiety reigns. This may cause some of us to starve ourselves for fear digestive upset will start, but for many more of us, it triggers cravings and urges us to binge on comfort food. It's no wonder that our insulin levels get fatigued, stress levels remain chronic, and the ability to regulate our moods greatly suffers.

How to Support Your Digestive System with Essential Oils

Preferred Essential Oils

PEPPERMINT (*Mentha piperita*)

- Reduces gas and bloating by relaxing smooth muscle spasms in colon
- Alleviates symptoms of occasional stomach upset and/or indigestion
- Alleviates discomfort from occasional gas and bloating

Aromatic Use

- Inhale straight from the bottle.
- Dilute and add 1 drop to palms, rub together, cup hands over nose, and inhale deeply.

Topical Use

- Dilute 1–2 drops with a carrier oil and rub over abdomen.
- Dilute 1–2 drops with a carrier oil and circle around belly button.
- Dilute 1–2 drops with a carrier oil and massage on the stomach.

GINGER (*Zingiber officinale*)

- Soothes digestive system and muscles to aid in healthy digestion
- Reduces occasional nausea and supports healthy digestive function
- Alleviates discomfort from occasional gas and bloating

Aromatic Use

- Inhale from the bottle before or during a long trip to alleviate motion sickness.
- Dilute and add 1 drop to palms, rub together, cup over nose, and inhale deeply to alleviate motion sickness.
- Add 3–4 drops to a diffuser.

Topical Use
- Dilute 1–2 drops with a carrier oil and warming massage into the abdomen.
- Dilute 1–2 drops with a carrier oil and rub around belly button.

Internal Use
- Add 1 drop to your morning green smoothie.

CARDAMOM (*Elettaria cardamomum*)

- Eases occasional digestive discomfort by soothing intestinal muscle contractions
- Alleviates bowel tension and looseness
- Calms and soothes digestive system, while having the same effect on body and mind

Aromatic Use
- Diffuse 3–4 drops.
- Dilute and add 1 drop to palms, rub together, cup over nose, and breathe deeply.

Topical Use
- Dilute 1–2 drops with a carrier oil and massage into abdomen.

CLOVE (*Eugenia caryophyllata*)

- Helps body to regulate systems during times of high stress or tension
- Has powerful immune-supporting properties and high levels of antioxidants to support overall wellness
- Supports healthy digestive and cardiovascular function by soothing and relaxing the body

Aromatic Use
- Diffuse 3–4 drops.
- Inhale from the bottle to alleviate occasional nausea and digestive discomfort.

Topical Use
- Dilute 1–2 drops with a carrier oil and massage into abdomen or over tense muscles.
- Add 1 diluted drop to toothpaste.

FENNEL (*Foeniculum vulgare*)

- Reduces stress and supports healthy digestive function
- Supports the liver and circulation while promoting a healthy metabolism
- Helps to combat sugar cravings that may lead to digestive discomfort

Aromatic Use

- Diffuse 3–4 drops.
- Dilute and add 1 drop to palms, rub together, cup over nose, and inhale deeply.

Topical Use

- Dilute 1–2 drops with a carrier oil and rub around belly button and stomach.
- Dilute 1–2 drops with a carrier oil and massage into abdomen.

Nicole's Story

Nicole was thirty-eight years old, an accountant and avid hiker, who came to me with complaints of a sluggish digestive system and occasional constipation. She was experiencing two to four bowel movements a week and always felt gassy and bloated. She also was feeling exhausted by 4 p.m., which she hadn't felt in the past, and began noticing excess weight around her belly despite vigorously hiking several times a week.

Nicole was experiencing estrogen dominance, slow digestion, and higher than normal levels of stress at work. **My recommendations were as follows:**

- Mindfully chewing her food, as the digestive process begins in your mouth, thanks to your saliva.

- A focus on eating whole foods such as green smoothies, vegetables, healthy fats, lean proteins, and gluten-free grains.
- For reducing stress at work, diffuse or inhale a combination of Bergamot, Lavender, and Frankincense essential oils, or the Zen Inhaler Blend (page 88).
- For digestive upset, use the Digestive Support Diffuser Blend (page 238) or the Belly Bliss Rollerball Blend (page 148).
- To reduce gas and bloating after each meal, use the Belly Bliss Rollerball Blend (page 148) before eating.
- Increased hydration with water, with Peppermint and Lemon essential oils in the afternoon to improve energy and gut motility.
- Fermented foods added to her diet to support a healthy gut microbiome and ease gas and bloating. Whole food probiotics are great for gut health.
- Adding digestive enzymes 15 to 30 minutes before a meal to aid in digestion.
- The 14-Day Rescue Plan to help reset her gut flora and boost her metabolism.

Within fifteen days, Nicole experienced more regular bowel movements. Her stress levels decreased at work and she told me she had more energy for her hikes after work. She lost five pounds on the 14-Day Rescue Plan and noticed that most of the weight came off around her midsection. Nicole also loved the way the oils supported her energy levels and digestion after her bigger meal. The bloating and gas disappeared once she started to use the oils regularly.

Essential Oil Blends

Aromatic Diffuser Blends

Rest and Digest Diffuser Blend

3 drops Lavender essential oil

2 drops Peppermint essential oil

Digestive Support Diffuser Blend

2 drops Lemon essential oil

1 drop Peppermint essential oil

1 drop Cardamom essential oil

1 drop Fennel essential oil

Digest and Uplift Diffuser Blend

2 drops Wild Orange essential oil

2 drops Ginger essential oil

1 drop Ylang Ylang essential oil

Aromatic Personal Inhaler Blends

Belly Blues Inhaler Blend

4 drops Ginger essential oil

4 drops Spearmint essential oil

3 drops Fennel essential oil

2 drops Lime essential oil

Travel Tamer Inhaler Blend

4 drops Peppermint essential oil

4 drops Ginger essential oil

3 drops Fennel essential oil

2 drops Cardamom essential oil

Cravings-Away Inhaler Blend

5 drops Wild Orange essential oil

4 drops Clove essential oil

2 drops Peppermint essential oil

2 drops Fennel essential oil

2 drops Lavender essential oil

Topical Rollerball Blends

Motion Sickness Rollerball Blend

10 drops Peppermint essential oil

5 drops Ginger essential oil

Carrier oil of choice

Add the essential oils to a 10 mL glass rollerball bottle and fill the rest with a carrier oil. Replace the rollerball and cap, and shake gently to blend. To use, apply before your trip as a preventative and then behind the ears every 15 to 20 minutes as needed until symptoms subside.

Overindulging Indigestion Rollerball Blend

10 drops Peppermint essential oil

10 drops Fennel essential oil

Carrier oil of choice

Add the essential oils to a 10 mL glass rollerball bottle and fill the rest with a carrier oil. Replace the rollerball and cap, and shake gently to blend. To use, apply down the esophageal area and circle in between the rib cage to reach the stomach. If the discomfort has gone lower, also circle around the belly button. Repeat every 15 to 20 minutes until distress subsides.

Self-Care Rituals for Digestive Issues

Remember that stress can be the biggest obstacle to a healthy digestive system, so be sure to refer to the de-stressing self-care rituals in Chapter 5. In addition, the suggestions for weight control in Chapter 8 and for improved sleep in Chapter 7, especially the Nighttime Self-Care Ritual, are also soothing and satisfying.

Digestive Massage Ritual

A soothing digestive massage can help keep you in tune with your body and also be a relaxing way to end your day. Choose the single essential oil or digestive blend that appeals to your senses the most. Starting around the belly button, apply a drop or two of the oil and begin to gently massage into your skin using an upward circular motion. Apply gentle pressure with the pads of your fingertips, circling to the right, for 10 to 15 slow strokes. This can also be repeated on your back, over your liver, and over your stomach depending on where your body needs it the most.

Enjoyable Eating Ritual

Though you may not realize it, we tend to eat too fast. Our bodies need time to complete all the digestive processes, but a stressful schedule can leave you running for fuel and eating on the way to the next disaster.

As soon as you start eating, saliva begins the digestive process before you've swallowed your first mouthful. The slower you chew, the more you will break down the food so that your digestive system can properly do its job. Always sit down to eat, which will encourage you to savor your food. Set a nice table and put your fork down between bites. Think about how your food tastes and what it does for your body. Make eating an enjoyable act for your body and mind, and your digestive system will thank you. Your brain pays as much attention to what you're eating as your stomach does!

CHAPTER 14

Toxicity

Life in the twenty-first century is driven by amazing techno-
logical advances that connect us on a global scale and make
so many tasks a breeze, but the flip side is the harm it does to our
planet—and to us, of course. One of the most tragic facts of our lives
is that we do not inhabit a clean world anymore. If you're thinking
that you buy organic produce and green cleaners, and use mostly
natural beauty products, you should be good, right? Sadly, the answer is no. The toxic assault is relentless and unavoidable, so even
a relatively healthy lifestyle can't make you immune. Anywhere
from 80,000 to 85,000 chemicals have been approved for use in
the United States, but only 200 of these have been subjected to
thorough testing, and many focusing on their impact only on adult
males in settings conducive to prolonged exposure. With the majority of these chemicals being unavoidable, transmitted through
the air, on land, and in groundwater, you need to know how to protect yourself.

One of my chores as a child was cleaning the bathrooms in our
house with harsh chemicals, and I soon began experiencing hor-
rific migraines each week after this job was done. There were no
organic, natural-based cleansers then, and all I knew was that the

household products that we used, and that everyone else used, made me sick.

As I mentioned earlier, I later learned that my lineage of hormone chaos is due in large part to my grandmother's being exposed to endocrine-disrupting chemicals when she was in her twenties. Fortunately, you can take many positive steps to reduce your toxic load and purify your environment. Starting now! Change what and how you eat; purge those harmful personal-care, beauty, and cleaning products and replace them with healthier, less-expensive, DIY versions. You won't believe the difference this can make in your overall vitality, and you will be amazed at the power of all-natural cleaning and the efficacy of all-natural personal-care products—especially when you add the power of essential oils.

The Why *Behind Toxicity*

Many people have no idea about how their toxic load affects their hormones, but I do because as a hormone expert, I have spent decades researching how chemicals affect women's hormones and their endocrine and reproductive systems. It's like a gigantic iceberg steadily growing underneath your body's surface—the result of decades of chemicals and toxins stressing your systems and vital organs. Your liver and kidneys can filter only so much of the toxins, and when they are overloaded, the chemicals wreak havoc from the inside out. Here are some terms you should know.

Toxic contaminant is something that contaminates a substance such as water or food, most commonly from chemicals, environmental threats, and radiation. Any substance with a consistent chemical composition is considered to be a chemical.

Chemicals are natural or synthetic substances that can potentially stress the body, most often found in environmental pollutants, processed food, xenoestrogens, and other common everyday products.

Radiation occurs when high-energy particles negatively influence cellular structures and DNA, the most common form provided by the sun.

Toxic load encompasses the quantity and effect these substances, which have accumulated over time, have on the body and the resulting stress placed on the body's systems and vital organs. Whatever can't be filtered naturally by the liver and kidneys causes damage until something is done to reverse the effects.

Our Body's Response to Toxins

Toxins invade from a variety of places, but direct exposure through the lungs, digestive system, and/or skin is by far the worst. Fortunately, our bodies are designed with defense mechanisms to filter out toxins: the mucous membranes in our mouths, noses, and throats and the powerful immune cells in our lungs. Although we can't always control the air we breathe or our environmental exposure, we *can* control our personal environments—what we expose our bodies to topically and physically, as well as what we consume.

Toxins You Ingest

Our food sources have been increasingly manipulated with harmful consequences, often by unscrupulous corporations that care more about their profits than our health. Many non-organic food sources are exposed to herbicides and pesticides. Science has shown that the more pesticides used, the more resistant those pests that bother these crops become, thereby negating the effectiveness of the very pesticides. Their solution? Use even more pesticides.

To avoid these foods, choose those labeled "certified organic," or shop at your local farmers' market or co-op. Additionally, consult the Environmental Working Group's website or an app to help you in making your food selections.

Another form of toxins you can unwittingly ingest are heavy metals such as mercury, aluminum, lead, nickel, and arsenic. Found

EWG'S Dirty Dozen and Clean 15

Each year, the Environmental Working Group (EWG) evaluates American produce, analyzing the testing done by the USDA, and makes recommendations to the general public. In 2017, they found that, in their samples, 70 percent of our common produce was contaminated with 178 different pesticides and residues, even after they were cleaned and peeled. The good news is that you can avoid most of these by buying organic from the group's Dirty Dozen list and choose regularly from the Clean 15 list.

Dirty Dozen

(Listed in order of most contaminated to least)

Strawberries	Pears
Spinach	Cherries
Nectarines	Tomatoes
Apples	Bell Peppers
Peaches	Potatoes
Celery	Hot Peppers (Bonus
Grapes	entry!)

Clean 15

(Listed from cleanest to a max of only four pesticides detected)

Sweet corn	Mangoes
Avocados	Eggplant
Pineapples	Honeydew melon
Cabbage	Kiwis
Onions	Cantaloupe
Frozen Sweet Peas	Cauliflower
Papayas	Grapefruit
Asparagus	

in the air, food, drinks, the metal fillings in your teeth, household cleaners, and even our drinking water, these heavy metals can cause major oxidative stress and damage on the cellular level, especially to your mitochondria. They can also displace important minerals and co-factors, deplete antioxidant levels, and act as endocrine disruptors, leading to hormone imbalance.

Toxins Generated in Your Body

Through the process of turning the food we eat into energy, we create oxidative by-products called *free radicals*. This is a perfectly normal process, but when your cells don't receive enough of the right nutrients, you can become deficient in the free-radical neutralizers you need, affecting your DNA and influencing the aging process while you can slowly develop chronic immune deficiencies and other illnesses such as cancer, diabetes, heart disease, and neurogenerative diseases. Excessive exercise, infection, or trauma can also upset the balance needed between antioxidants and free radicals that keeps our bodies functioning. Eating lots of antioxidant-rich foods is key to keeping free radicals at bay.

In addition, millions of Americans whose diets are not properly balanced have sluggish digestion due to toxins in the digestive tract. As described in the previous chapter, disease-causing inflammation begins in the gut, so it's extremely important to eat a lot of fiber-rich foods so you can eliminate allergens and toxins in your food as quickly as possible.

Last but certainly not least, infectious agents such as bacteria, viruses, mold, parasites, yeast, and other organisms can make a home in your body under certain conditions. Many of these bugs thrive in the digestive tract when it's overly acidic and not colonized by enough healthy bacteria. Factor in the toxins from food as well as from pollutants, heavy metals, and stressors, and you can lower your immune system and impact your gut health. Maintaining a proper microbiome and healthy body is your best defense, and will allow your body to process those toxins so you can get rid of them.

Environmental Toxins—Outside and in Your Home

In addition to internal free radicals, external influences such as cigarette smoke, industrial solvents, ozone pollution, pharmaceuticals, pesticides, pollutants in the environment, and radiation can trigger the same effect, and make you very sick.

Although we may think that we are protected *inside* our homes, the Environmental Protection Agency (EPA) has reported that the air inside our homes is typically two to five times *more* polluted than the air outside! You're inhaling toxins from cleaning products, air fresheners, paints, carpets, furniture, smoke from cooking, dirty filters in air conditioners, and dry cleaning, among other sources. This is especially egregious in newer buildings that might be more energy efficient, but that don't have good ventilation or windows that open all the way. In fact, a new illness known as sick building syndrome is attributed to many office buildings and hotels where the same air is recirculated over and over again, contaminating their residents.

My husband and I live in an older home, and are lucky to have gorgeous French doors in our bedroom that fully open out to a courtyard and avocado tree. I work in front of them all the time, and they're always open, as are our windows, when the weather permits, for the best possible air circulation. Our diffusers are also going so essential oils can rid the air of toxins, thanks to their antimicrobial properties that can zap airborne toxins in thirty to sixty minutes. Even though the environment outside is beyond our control, our internal home environment can be protected by diffusing high-quality essential oils and making our own products.

You're going to love the options in this chapter for purifying your home. Start small, replacing one product at a time, and experiment with scents and natural ingredients to find the best combinations you like. You will be amazed at the money you'll save and how easy it is to keep your house in top condition with just a small arsenal of ingredients!

Environmental Toxins—Personal Care Products

Women in particular are at severe risk for overexposure to endocrine-disrupting chemicals (EDCs) owing to the personal-care and beauty products we love. The average woman uses around twelve products daily on her skin, including roughly 126 different ingredients, but 90 percent of those ingredients have *never* been researched for safety by any publicly accountable institution like the FDA. Even more frightening is that, since our skin absorbs anything applied to it, a woman can absorb five pounds of toxins per year just from her beauty-care routine.

It is shocking that the FDA and cosmetic corporations continue to insist that, if used in small daily amounts, these chemicals pose no immediate risk. Strong scientific evidence links dangerous toxins and synthetics in these personal-care products to reproductive disorders, autoimmune disorders, allergies, and even cancer. Preservatives like parabens and phthalates (which are banned in many countries) used in fragrances, cosmetics, and hair-care products can even be detected in breast milk and body tissues.

Being label savvy with your personal-care products will help to protect you, but manufacturers are very good at providing misleading information. The only mandates are that drug-like ingredients be listed in a box marked "Active Ingredients," and other ingredients are listed starting with the highest proportion first. If you don't recognize an ingredient, look up some of the complicated chemical names on the packaging; some of them sound toxic but are actually safe and effective, such as vitamin derivatives. But others will not be.

Because it is so challenging to decipher these labels and assess what's toxic or not, I highly recommend making as many of your own personal-care products as possible. Not only will they be good for you, especially when enriched by essential oils that will also make them smell delicious, but they will also cost a fraction of their store-bought counterparts. I tell women they should be able to eat most of the ingredients in their personal-care products. Of course, I don't recommend actually eating them, but you *should* be able to! Minimal amounts of pronounceable ingredients are always safer than questionable and unrecognizable ones.

Your Hormones and Toxicity

What do all these toxins and chemicals do to our hormones? They're endocrine disruptors (EDs), which alter normal hormonal function by blocking and binding hormone receptors while negatively affecting the brain, reproduction, and metabolic development. In women, chemical preservatives and plastics such as BPA, parabens, and phthalates can alter reproductive development and fertility, as well as be the cause of early onset of menopause. Xenoestrogens, found in food and in personal-care products, mimic the estrogen you produce, as mentioned in Chapter 9, and can cause estrogen dominance, as well as other endocrine and bodily issues. In men, these chemicals are linked to male infertility, genital deformities, and even cancer.

These are the most common EDs and their effects on hormones:

Arsenic
> **Found in:** food and drinking water; tobacco
> **Toxic identification:** carcinogen; endocrine disruptor

Atrazine
> **Found in:** crops such as corn, sorghum, sugarcane, macadamia nuts, and beans; playgrounds, athletic fields, lawns, and evergreen trees; drinking water
> **Toxic identification:** herbicide; endocrine disruptor

Bisphenol-A (BPA)

The trade journal *Environmental Health Perspectives* reviewed studies from 2007 to 2013 dealing with BPA, linking it to reproductive and developmental problems in animals as well as human fetuses and newborns. They labeled BPA as a reproductive toxin, in addition to an endocrine-disrupting threat to a variety of bodily systems.

> **Found in:** plastics
>
> **Toxic identification:** xenoestrogen

Dioxin and Furan

A by-product of industrial processes.

> **Found in:** throughout the environment; in our food supply, mainly in the fatty tissue of animals
>
> **Toxic identification:** carcinogen, endocrine disruptor

Fire Retardants

> **Found in:** building materials, electronics, furniture, textiles (especially children's pajamas)
>
> **Toxic identification:** endocrine disruptor; imitate thyroid hormones

Glycol Ethers

> **Found in:** paints, cleaning products, brake fluid, cosmetics
>
> **Toxic identification:** endocrine disruptor

Lead

> **Found in:** batteries, ammunition, old pipes, old paint, caulking, and ceramics
>
> **Toxic identification:** endocrine disruptor, especially detrimental to HPA axis; potential carcinogen

Mercury

Burning coal releases it into the atmosphere.

> **Found in:** in air and oceans; seafood contaminated with methylmercury
>
> **Toxic identification:** endocrine disruptor

Organophosphate Pesticides

Found in: pesticides

Toxic identification: endocrine disruptor, specifically testosterone levels and thyroid levels; carcinogen

Perchlorate (often called perc)

Found in: dry cleaning; produce, milk, and water; rocket fuel; matches and flares; fertilizers; hypochlorite bleach

Toxic identification: thyroid disruptor

Perfluorinated chemicals (PFCs)

Found in: nonstick cookware, waterproof coatings for furniture, some food packaging, and in other industries

Toxic identification: endocrine disruptor, especially thyroid and sex hormone levels; potential carcinogen

Phthalates

Found in: plastic food containers, children's toys, plastic wrap made from PVC (recycling label #3), personal care products (listed as "fragrance"), and hundreds of products from vinyl flooring and adhesives to detergents and medical tubing

Toxic identification: endocrine disruptor; potential carcinogen

Emotional Triggers

Stress continues to be the biggest emotional trigger for many of us, especially when we increase our knowledge of our toxic load, as well as the threat of environmental toxins. When toxins begin to affect your hormonal balance, it's even harder to control your moods and feel grounded. Following the tips in Chapter 5 to reduce the stress in your life will be a great start, but the biggest change will come from revamping the toxin-containing products in your home. You can improve your mood from the inside out and the outside in.

How to Reduce Toxicity with Essential Oils

Preferred Essential Oils

CILANTRO (*Coriandrum sativum*)

- Powerful detoxifier when taken internally to support healthy digestion
- Supports healthy immune and nervous system function
- Rids your home of unwanted odors and cleanses the air

Aromatic Use

- Diffuse 2 drops with 2 drops of Grapefruit or Lemon.
- Diffuse 3–4 drops.

Topical Use

- Dilute 1–2 drops with a carrier oil and massage where needed.
- Dilute 1–2 drops with a carrier oil massage over the abdomen.

GRAPEFRUIT (*Citrus × paradisi*)

- Uplifts moods and emotions while easing anxiety and stressful feelings
- Helps flush out built-up toxins from the body and supports a healthy metabolism when taken internally
- Enhances motivation, energizes the body, and curbs cravings

Aromatic Use

- Diffuse 3–4 drops.
- Add 1 drop to a cotton ball and insert in needed areas to deodorize and purify.

Topical Use

- Dilute 1–2 drops with a carrier oil with organic Jojoba oil and apply as a spot treatment for blemishes.
- Dilute 1–2 drops with a carrier oil and massage into the body; focus on the neck and shoulders.
- Add to your DIY body washes and scrubs.

WARNING: Citrus oils are naturally phototoxic, so avoid direct sun exposure for at least 12 hours after topical application.

JUNIPER BERRY (*Juniperus communis*)

- Cleanses and purifies the air
- Promotes healthy kidney and urinary tract function
- Natural detoxifier with a calming and grounding effect on the mind and body

Aromatic Use

- Diffuse 3–4 drops.
- Diffuse 2 drops with 2 drops Bergamot, Grapefruit, or Lemon.

Topical Use

- Dilute 1–2 drops with a carrier oil and massage directly into skin to tone and reduce blemishes.
- Add 1–2 drops to a Detoxing and Purifying Clay Face Mask (page 264) and apply.

LAVENDER (*Lavandula angustifolia*)

- Calms and relaxes the mind and body from stress
- Aids in effective and restful sleep to allow the body to reset
- Soothes minor skin irritations

Aromatic Use

- Diffuse 3–4 drops.
- Add a few drops to your pillow or bedclothes.
- Add a few drops to your potpourri or on the inside cardboard of a toilet paper roll.

Topical Use

- Dilute 1–2 drops with a carrier oil and massage into pulse points.
- Dilute 1–2 drops with a carrier oil and apply to the bottoms of your feet.
- Add to any of your DIY personal care recipes to soothe and calm irritated skin.
- Add 3–4 drops to ½ cup Epsom salts dissolved in a warm bath.

LEMON (*Citrus lemon*)

- Cleanses the body from built-up toxins while uplifting mood
- Effective hard-surface cleaner

- Boosts the respiratory and digestive systems with antioxidant power

Aromatic Use
- Diffuse 3–4 drops.
- Dilute and place 1 drop in palms, rub together, cup over nose, and practice deep breathing.
- Diffuse 3 drops Lemon with 1 drop Peppermint.

Topical Use
- Dilute 1–2 drops with a carrier oil and apply to your chest to break up mucus and aid the body in releasing toxins. Follow with diluted Peppermint for respiratory support.
- Use in your homemade hand soap as a natural degreaser.
- Add to your own exfoliating scrub.

Internal Use
- Add 1–2 drops to 2 cups water in a stainless steel or glass bottle and sip throughout the day.
- Add 1 drop to your daily green smoothie.

WARNING: Citrus oils are naturally phototoxic, so be sure to dilute and avoid direct sun exposure for at least 12 hours after topical application.

ROSEMARY (*Rosmarinus officinalis*)
- Improves mental recall, focus, and cognition
- Enhances digestion and internal organ function as well as healthy respiratory function
- Reduces tension and helps the body to de-stress from nervous energy and fatigue

Aromatic Use
- Diffuse 3–4 drops.
- Diffuse 2 drops with 1 drop Peppermint.

Topical Use
- Add 3–4 drops to ½ cup Epsom salts dissolved in a warm bath.
- Add 2–3 drops to your shampoo, conditioner, or hair care products.

- Dilute 1–2 drops with a carrier oil and massage into your body; especially effective when combined with Peppermint. For a more relaxing massage, combine with Lavender.

PEPPERMINT (*Mentha piperita*)

- Opens airways naturally and promotes healthy respiratory function
- Enlivens the senses and piques mental focus
- Supports healthy digestive function including vital organs clogged from toxic load

Aromatic Use

- Diffuse 2 drops of Peppermint with 2 drops of a citrus essential oil.
- Add 1 drop to palms, rub together, cup over nose, and practice deep breathing.

Topical Use

- Dilute 1–2 drops with a carrier oil.
- Add 5 drops to a 2-ounce glass spray bottle and mist your face.

WARNING: Peppermint contains menthol and is a cooling oil. In case of cross-contamination, always dilute with a carrier oil or a vegetable oil, not water!

Wendy's Story

Wendy, a forty-five-year-old beauty consultant and esthetician, came to me with severe night sweats, low libido, and migraine headaches one or two times a week. She also experienced irritability and mood swings throughout the month, and told me that she'd had migraines for over five years, but they were becoming worse. She assumed her hormones were imbalanced, but couldn't figure out what was going on since she wasn't in menopause yet.

Wendy was experiencing estrogen dominance along with perimenopausal symptoms and increased toxic load. **My recommendations were as follows:**

- The 14-Day Rescue Plan to detoxify the body and improve gut health.
- For head and neck tension, Peppermint, Lavender, and Frankincense essential oils.
- For reducing toxic load, she should go through her office and home and remove any toxic skin-care and beauty-care products. She should discontinue the use of toxic skin-care and makeup items.
- For mood support, the Happy Bliss Inhaler Blend (page 203) and Energize Your Mood Inhaler Blend (page 203) to use throughout the day. And added Bergamot and Lavender to lesson irritability and stress.
- A "hot flash" spray of Peppermint, Clary Sage, and Lavender essential oils on her bed stand anytime she experienced night sweats.
- To support organ detoxification, increased water intake with lemon juice and Lemon essential oil in the morning and afternoon, or make a detox water.

- Supplements: multivitamin, 200 mg S-acetylated glutathione, dandelion tea at night, and 500 mg milk thistle.
- Prepare cleaning products with essential oils and natural ingredients and remove plastic from the home.

After seven weeks, Wendy told me she'd only had one migraine, fewer night sweats, and had lost five pounds. She removed all the plastic and toxic items from her home. She replaced the skin-care products at work with an organic brand and her clients loved the change. Wendy noticed that her mood significantly improved. "My overall mood feels so much lighter and more joyful!" she told me. "I had no idea the negative impact my skin-care and makeup products were having on my body and hormones. Even though it was hard to make over all of my products, I am so grateful that I did. I can feel the difference when my body is clear of toxins."

Essential Oil Blends

Aromatic Diffuser Blends

Enliven and Focus Diffuser Blend

3 drops Grapefruit or Lemon essential oil
2 drops Peppermint essential oil

Invigorate and Deodorize Diffuser Blend

3 drops Grapefruit essential oil
2 drops Peppermint essential oil
2 drops Lime essential oil

Cleanse the Air Diffuser Blend

2 drops Grapefruit essential oil

2 drops Lemon essential oil

1 drop Melaleuca essential oil

1 drop Rosemary essential oil

Breathe and Receive Diffuser Blend

2 drops Eucalyptus essential oil

2 drops Peppermint essential oil

1 drop Melaleuca essential oil

1 drop Lemon essential oil

Aromatic Personal Inhaler Blends

Allergen Support Inhaler Blend

5 drops Lavender essential oil

5 drops Lemon essential oil

5 drops Peppermint essential oil

Immune Support Inhaler Blend

4 drops Melaleuca essential oil

4 drops Rosemary essential oil

4 drops Frankincense essential oil

3 drops Lemon essential oil

Deep Breathing Inhaler Blend

4 drops Peppermint essential oil

4 drops Eucalyptus essential oil

3 drops Lavender essential oil

2 drops Lemon essential oil

Topical Rollerball Blends

Love Your Liver Massage Rollerball Blend

5 drops Geranium essential oil
5 drops Fennel essential oil
3 drops Grapefruit essential oil
3 drops Ginger essential oil
2 drops Rosemary essential oil
Carrier oil of choice

Add the essential oils to a 10 mL glass rollerball bottle and top with a carrier oil of your choice. Replace the rollerball and cap, and shake to mix. Apply to the liver and gently massage into the body.

Endocrine Support Detox Rollerball Blend

10 drops Grapefruit essential oil
8 drops Geranium essential oil
5 drops Juniper Berry essential oil
2 drops Cilantro essential oil

Add the essential oils to a 10 mL glass rollerball bottle and top with a carrier oil of your choice. Replace the rollerball and cap, and shake to mix. Apply to your soles before bedtime.

Internal Uses

Berry Boost Antioxidant Water Infusion

½ cup organic blueberries
½ cup organic blackberries
½ cup organic raspberries
½ cup organic strawberries
½ cup organic cherries, halved and pitted
¼ small organic red beet, peeled and chopped
1 quart plus 2 cups filtered water
2 drops Lemon essential oil

Combine the fruits, beet, and 2 cups water in a blender and process until smooth, approximately 1 minute. Pour the blend through a fine-mesh sieve into a 2-quart pitcher, then add the essential oil and stir. Pour in the remaining water and then refrigerate the infusion for at least 30 minutes. Serve chilled or over ice.

Renewing Detox Water Infusion

½ cup organic blueberries
2 drops Grapefruit essential oil
1 organic lemon, sliced into rounds
½ cup organic cucumber, sliced
1½ quarts filtered water

Muddle the blueberries and essential oil in a small glass bowl. Add the mixture to a 2-quart pitcher along with the lemon and cucumber slices. Pour in the water and refrigerate for 3 to 5 hours before serving. (Can refrigerate for up to 3 days.)

Essential Oil Blends for Home Use

For more green cleaning and personal-care recipes, check out my book *Smart Mom's Guide to Essential Oils*. These are the top ingredients you will need to make your own products:

- Baking soda
- Citric acid
- Distilled white vinegar
- Essential oils: Lemon, Grapefruit, Melaleuca, Lavender, Wild Orange, Eucalyptus, Peppermint
- Kosher salt
- Liquid castile soap (such as Dr. Bronner's)
- Vegetable glycerin

- Washing soda (sodium carbonate or soda ash)
- Witch hazel or rubbing alcohol

Kitchen, Bathroom, and Laundry Cleaning

All-Purpose Cleaner

1 cup distilled white vinegar

2 cups warm water

10 drops citrus essential oil (Lemon, Grapefruit, Wild Orange)

10 drops Melaleuca essential oil

Note: Other EO combinations include 10 drops Lemon + 10 drops Lavender, or 7 drops each Peppermint, Melaleuca, and Citrus

Combine all the ingredients in a 16-ounce glass spray bottle. Shake and spritz to use, and then wipe clean with a microfiber cloth. This works for the majority of hard surfaces, or for tougher areas, leave the solution on for 5 to 15 minutes before wiping clean. For deep cleaning, sprinkle baking soda on the surface before spraying.

Glass Cleaner

2 cups distilled water

2 tablespoons white vinegar

1 tablespoon witch hazel or rubbing alcohol

5 drops citrus essential oil (ex: Wild Orange, Lemon, Lime, and Grapefruit)

Combine all the ingredients in a 16-ounce glass spray bottle and shake well. Spritz on windows, mirrors, and glass surfaces, and then wipe down with a microfiber cloth. (Keeps up to 3 months when stored properly.)

Scrubbing Paste

¾ rounded cup baking soda

¼ cup liquid castile soap

1 tablespoon water
1 tablespoon distilled white vinegar
5–10 drops Lemon essential oil (or citrus oil of choice)

Combine all the ingredients into a paste in a glass jar. To use, apply over area and let sit for 15 minutes. Gently scrub with a sponge or microfiber cloth before wiping clean. (Store any extra in an airtight glass container.)

Dishwasher Detergent

1 cup washing soda
¼ cup citric acid
¼ cup kosher salt
Essential oils of choice

Mix all the ingredients in an airtight glass jar. To use, add 1 to 2 tablespoons to your dishwasher and wash as normal. Add vinegar in the rinse compartment as a booster or in place of a chemical rinse aid.

Laundry Detergent

1 cup washing soda
1 cup borax
1 bar castile soap, grated (scent of your choice)
Essential oils of choice

Add the washing soda and borax to the grated castile soap and mix. Store in an airtight glass jar. If the scent isn't as strong as you would like, add a few drops of essential oils. To use, add 1 tablespoon to your HE (high efficiency) washing machine. For extra cleaning power, add distilled white vinegar to the prewash cycle or soak towels and other hard-to-clean items with vinegar and water before washing.

Stain Remover

1 cup distilled white vinegar
12 drops Lemon essential oil

Combine the ingredients in an 8-ounce glass spray bottle. To use, shake and spritz each time, let sit for 5 to 10 minutes, and then wash immediately.

Personal-Care Blends

When blended with the right carrier oils, essentials oils are wonderful for soothing the skin and supporting cellular regeneration, as well as for toning and tightening, reducing blemishes and wrinkles, and smoothing dry, chapped skin. These essential oils have specific properties that will support the health of your overall body, especially your skin and hair:

- **For anti-aging properties**: Frankincense, Lavender, Neroli
- **For healthy complexion**: Helichrysum, Melaleuca, Rose, Frankincense
- **For common skin irritations**: Geranium combined with Lavender
- **For sensitive skin**: Frankincense, Lavender, Melaleuca, Roman Chamomile
- **For toning and purifying**: All citrus oils
- **For strong and healthy hair**: Cedarwood, Geranium, Lavender, Rosemary, Peppermint

Experiment with different essential oils to see which work best for your skin. I like to alternate among Sandalwood, Helichrysum, Rose, Jasmine, Orange, and Geranium. If the following cream is too rich for your face, you can use it for your hands and feet instead to soothe dry, cracked skin. Essential oils to consider for hand and foot creams are Peppermint, Rose Geranium, Calendula, Lemon, and Eucalyptus.

Clear Complexion Blemish Roller Blend

10 drops Melaleuca essential oil
7 drops Lavender essential oil
5 drops Geranium essential oil

3 drops Rosemary essential oil
Jojoba oil

In a 10 mL glass rollerball bottle, combine the essential oils and fill the rest of the way with jojoba oil. Replace the rollerball top and cap, and shake gently to blend. Apply after cleansing your face morning and night by rubbing your finger on the rollerball and gently dabbing the blend on problem areas.

Essential Oil Hair Growth and Repair Conditioner

Geranium will strengthen and protect your hair from the excess heat of tools such as blow dryers and curling irons, while Rosemary stimulates hair follicles and enhances growth. Melaleuca protects from scalp dryness, while Lavender soothes the scalp and Peppermint provides a refreshing tingle.

1½ cups distilled water
3 tablespoons raw organic apple cider vinegar (such as Bragg's)
6 drops Rosemary essential oil
5 drops Geranium essential oil
3 drops Lavender essential oil
3 drops Peppermint essential oil
3 drops Melaleuca essential oil

Add all the ingredients to an 8-ounce glass spray bottle. Shake the bottle gently before using and apply to roots and work into hair.

Oatmeal-Lemon Skin Exfoliating Scrub

¼ cup organic oatmeal, ground to a powder
Distilled water (enough to make a paste)
5 drops Lemon essential oil

Add the oatmeal to a glass bowl and add water a bit at a time until you have a paste. Add the Lemon essential oil and mix well. Rub in circular motions into your skin to naturally exfoliate, being careful to avoid sensitive areas. Allow to rest on the skin for 10 to 15 minutes to penetrate and soften, then gently rinse off with warm water. Pat your skin dry with a soft towel or microfiber cloth. Be sure to moisturize afterward. WARNING: Citrus oils are naturally phototoxic, so avoid direct sun exposure for at least 12 hours after using this scrub.

Detoxing and Purifying Clay Face Mask

2 teaspoons Bentonite clay (for a thicker mask, add ½ teaspoon more)

2 teaspoons organic apple cider vinegar (such as Bragg's)

1 drop Frankincense essential oil

1 drop Lavender essential oil

1 drop Melaleuca essential oil

1 drop Juniper Berry essential oil

Combine the clay and vinegar in a glass bowl, mixing with a silicone spoon. (Do NOT use metal, as it will make it less effective.) Add the essential oils and mix again. Apply to clean skin, massaging in your face while avoiding the eyes and mouth. Allow to dry for 5 to 15 minutes; it will begin to feel tight as it dries, but should not burn or itch at all. Be sure to rinse with warm water and follow with a moisturizer. If any irritation occurs, wash off immediately and then moisturize with a carrier oil, like jojoba or coconut.

Foaming Hand Soap

1½ cups distilled water

2 tablespoons liquid castile soap

1 teaspoon vegetable glycerin

½ teaspoon coconut or sweet almond oil

Essential oils of choice (I recommend a Citrus/Lavender combo for the kitchen, and immune-boosting EOs for the bathroom, such as Cinnamon, Clove, and Wild Orange)

In a foaming soap dispenser, add the water, leaving room at the top. Then add the soap, glycerin, oil, and essential oils. Close tightly and lightly tip upside down and return to proper position to mix. If you shake it too much, it will bubble inside. To use, pump into your hand and wash as you normally would.

Self-Care Rituals for Toxicity

Monthly Clean-Out Ritual

Every month, I recommend picking an area to examine for chemicals lurking in your household. Then, make your own products or purchase ones that are safer. Start with your cleaning cabinet and trash anything that isn't all-natural. Next month, take a look at your personal-care products. Then, a month later, tackle your beauty products. Eventually, you will replace your entire home with healthy, hormone-safe solutions. As always, essential oils are the best way to amp up your arsenal and keep your repertoire personalized for your needs. Experimentation is half the fun!

Oil-Pulling Ritual

Oil pulling, also known by its Ayurvedic names, *gundusha* or *kavala*, has been utilized for thousands of years in holistic medicine. It is an amazing addition to your overall health and wellness arsenal, as it can cleanse and detoxify your mouth in a way that traditional oral hygiene techniques can't, leaving you with less tooth decay, better breath, healthier gums, and whiter teeth. It can also reduce inflammation, soothe a dry throat, boost your immune system, and even reduce acne. It's best performed first thing in the morning on an empty stomach.

Use a high-quality cold-pressed organic coconut oil, as it contains easily digestible, fat-soluble vitamins and other nutrients. Other people prefer olive oil, sesame, sunflower, or palm oil. The actual act is simple, but it takes some getting used to. Place 1 tablespoon of oil in your mouth. It will immediately liquify and you can begin to swish and pull it through your teeth and around your mouth. It doesn't need to be vigorous (as with mouthwash), but it does need to be consistent and prolonged. Do this for *20* minutes. It may take several tries to get used to the sensation of oil in your mouth, but trust me . . . it's worth it! After 20 minutes, spit out all the coconut oil, which rids your body of the toxins it has picked up. Rinse your mouth well with warm salt water and then brush your teeth.

Repeat this once a day for two weeks, and then take a break for several weeks before resuming. For an extra boost once you get used to the process, try adding a drop of Lemon or Peppermint essential oil to the coconut oil before putting it in your mouth.

Work Up a Good Sweat Ritual

Regular exercise helps your body to sweat and release toxins naturally while keeping your lungs in top condition to filter airborne toxins. Always be sure to hydrate before, during, and after exercise, as your kidneys' and liver's ability to transform toxins into water-soluble chemicals to excrete is hampered when you're dehydrated.

Dry Skin Brushing Ritual

For an amazingly easy and fulfilling daily ritual, dry brushing in the morning is fantastic. Using a dry skin brush, work in circular motions to gently massage the skin, starting with your feet and pulling up toward the heart. You can then move to the palms and pull in to the heart. On the stomach and armpits, use a clockwise motion and then move to your back and abdomen. I recommend repeating ten strokes for each area.

In addition to stimulating the lymphatic system to support the removal of toxins, dry brushing will also help slough off dead skin cells, cleansing your pores and leaving your skin smooth. Try diffusing a calming essential oil blend as you brush, taking your time to enjoy each stroke. Finish by showering to remove what you've sloughed off.

Detox Bath Soak Rituals

A weekly detox bath soak is a simple and calming ritual that can help your body to release unwanted toxins while relaxing and recharging. Usually, I reserve a special time in the evening at the end of the week to take my bath, and make it a special occasion by diffusing my special oils, playing my favorite calming tunes on my phone, and closing my eyes during my soak.

Detox and Relax Bath Soak

½ cup sea salt
½ cup Epsom salts or magnesium flakes
¼ cup baking soda
½ cup apple cider vinegar
4 drops Rosemary essential oil
4 drops Grapefruit essential oil
1 drop Ginger essential oil

Fill the bathtub with hot water. Mix the sea salt, Epsom salts, and baking soda in a small glass bowl. Add the dry mix and apple cider vinegar to the bath water and swirl with your hand to mix and dissolve. Blend the essential oils in the glass bowl, then add to the bath water, swirling to combine. Breathe deeply and soak no longer than 20 minutes. Rinse off the remaining salt on your body in the shower and moisturize well. Visualize all of your stressors washing down the drain as you continue to practice deep breathing.

PART III

The 14-Day Rescue Plan to Jump-Start Your Hormonal Health

If you had asked me ten years ago what I did to keep myself healthy and my hormones functioning at optimal levels, I would have said, "I go to the gym for one hour four or five times a week. Sure, I try to eat well (but have to admit I indulge my cravings for York Peppermint Patties at 4 p.m. every day). I drink two to three cups of coffee every day because I love it and can't live without it. I buy lots of vitamins, but maybe once in a while I forget to take them—my bad! I use whatever shampoo is on sale in the drugstore. Oh, and I work as hard as I possibly can until I collapse into bed (and then have a hard time going to sleep)."

Now, my schedule is *completely* different. A savory green smoothie and the supplements I need for breakfast every day? Check. Gratitude journaling and mindful breathing? You bet. A hike outside or high-intensity interval training at least five times a week? Wouldn't miss it. Fresh, simple, delicious meals, low in sugar and high in flavor? Of course. Nontoxic skin-care products that I love to make myself, that have given me the best skin and hair of my life? What a treat! Essential oils by my side all day long? Well, what do you think?!

All these activities have become second nature to me. I *never* thought they would—but they keep me healthy, vibrant, energized when I need to be, and relaxed when it's time to wind down, so I can't ever imagine going back to my former bad habits. My hormone chaos has been completely tamed by simple, effective home remedies, real food, and real exercise.

Here's the thing: I am *not* a different person. In terms of personality, I am the same woman I was a decade ago—but what did change was my determination to do the work I knew I needed to do to finally take care of myself the way I deserved to be taken care of.

I created the 14-Day Rescue Plan to give your body the jolt it needs to balance your hormones quickly and effectively, and show you how incorporating all the good habits you've read about in this book, especially in the previous chapter, will drastically improve your health. The plan consists of incorporating self-care techniques, rituals, and essential oils to help you reset your hormones. This is where the work comes in, because you have to listen to your body in order to know what it needs the most. By identifying the areas where your body needs work, you can begin to select the routines and rituals that make the most sense for you from Part II. I recommend marking them with a sticky-note flag so that you can easily reference them. Then, you can begin to work them into your daily routine—your morning and evening routines, as well as pitstops throughout the day for balance. If something doesn't work for you, stop and swap it for something else.

Before beginning your 14-Day Rescue Plan, we need to firm up your foundation as well. Let's take a good, hard look at nutrition first, then exercise, and revisit stress management, eliminating the toxins and adding self-care routines. Success will come from using the Five Pillars for a Foundational Lifestyle presented in Chapter 15 as a guide to incorporating the self-care rituals that will help you create your individualized plan. These rituals will eventually become the habits that support you in your 14-Day Rescue Plan and beyond!

The next step is the addition of the 14-Day Rescue Meal Plan, which supports the other changes you have made. When you begin the meal plan, you will have already laid a firm foundation and have begun implementing the self-care routines and rituals for your hormonal rescue. You will not believe how well your body will respond when you tie everything together. Sure, there will be bumps along the way, but you can do it. Your body needs you to go all in and find yourself again. I'm right here with you to support you all the way.

The 8 Steps of the 14-Day Rescue Plan

1. Mark your routines and rituals with sticky-note flags. Rank them in order of importance based on your individual needs. Create a checklist for each of the following: morning routine, evening routine, stress management, and daily habits. Feel free to add more rituals per pillar or section as needed.

2. Create your essential-oils diary and your food journal to track how each oil, blend, and meal treats your body.

3. Read Chapter 15, making notes on the Five Pillars for how to firm up your foundation.

4. Begin incorporating the foundation-firming routines and the morning and evening rituals to discover what works best for you for one week.

5. Prepare for the 14-Day Rescue Meal Plan by shopping ahead and ensuring that you have all ingredients needed.

6. Clear your calendar. Be sure that you have two free weeks without added stress or travel, and get ready to start!

7. For 14 days, follow the 14-Day Rescue Meal Plan with your daily rituals and self-care routines. Note your successes and pitfalls in your food journal, your mood and bodily responses in your essential-oils diary, and your praises in your gratitude journal.

8. Review your journals and diary and see how you feel. Tweak according to your individual needs, then take a look at Chapter 18 for the Refresh and Replenish.

Let's get started!

Overwhelmed by the Steps? No Problem! Check Out Our Beginner's Guide Until You Figure Out What Works the Best for You!

Self-Care Rituals for Beginners

MORNING

Apply Superwoman Rollerball Blend

Shower Ritual with Awaken or Abundance Spritz

Drink 16 ounces of water with lemon

Green Smoothie and supplements

Gratitude journal (diffuse Frankincense or Wild Orange)

5 minutes of Move Your Body Ritual

PLAN THE DAY

Drink 6–8 cups water

Breathe-on-the-Hour Ritual

30 minutes of Move Your Body Ritual

Healthy Food Plan

EVENING

Prepare Your Sleep Environment

Mirror and Positive Affirmations Rituals

Wind Down to Sleep Ritual

CHAPTER 15

The Five Pillars of a Foundational Lifestyle

Before you dive into the 14-Day Rescue Plan, make sure you have the foundation to support these changes. As discussed in Part I, your body cannot do what it needs to do with so little to build upon. If your foundation is shaky, then the 14-Day Rescue Plan will not have the phenomenal effect on your overall health that it can have. The plan has the potential to help you reset your hormonal health, but you have to do some work ahead of time.

That's where the Five Pillars can be your guide. Each represents a core component that will help you strengthen your body's foundation so that your efforts to balance your hormones with essential oils can truly take hold and build you back up again. In this chapter, you will learn the steps to take to set that foundation so you will find success as a result of the 14-Day Rescue Plan. Do you have to do everything I have suggested? No, you don't have to, but you should examine the suggestions and see what works best for your needs. No one person's plan will look like anyone else's because this is all about you. Your heritage and your body make you a unique individual, so you need to feed your individual needs by setting your foundation and building upon it to reset your hormonal needs.

I recommend reading about the Five Pillars first, then going back to see which habits you need to incorporate initially. Chapter 16 is then a suggestion guide for getting the most from your Five Pillars, but again, feel free to adjust it according to your own needs. The same goes for the 14-Day Rescue Meal Plan—if there is a recipe you don't like, feel free to substitute any of the other recipes or substitute an ingredient with another healthy option. It's all about what works for you within the guidelines I've detailed. Everything here has a reason and a purpose, but the bigger overall purpose is for you to learn what works for you and to make the changes that fit your lifestyle so that you experience success!

Pillar #1—Nutrition

The Break-Ups

For the 14-Day Rescue Plan to be successful, it's time to get real about ending any relationships that have been abusing your body. Sugar, gluten, processed foods, and caffeine are the biggest offenders in our modern diet, and you've got to eliminate them beforehand. Once you begin the 14-Day Rescue Meal Plan, you will also eliminate dairy and red meat. Why? Because these foods cause inflammation and may be driving some of your symptoms. And, as you know, sugar also causes insulin spikes that lead to excess fat storage. It also affects your cortisol levels, which in turn affect your estrogen and progesterone levels. Gluten creates an inflammatory response in your thyroid. Coffee revs up those adrenal hormones. Red meat is loaded with female hormones that you definitely do not need to be ingesting, which can create estrogen dominance.

If you don't start now, your body will face too drastic a shock when you begin the 14-Day Rescue Plan and will leave you crumpled in the wake. I want you to succeed in this process, and I know that going cold turkey on these items will make you feel horrible at first. It will cause withdrawal, cravings, and digestive distress like you've never before experienced. And you will give up. I don't want that for you. Remember that when the fourteen days are over, you can begin reintroducing these foods one at a time, which will allow you to identify potential triggers and food items that harm your health.

So, let's discuss the *why* for the break-ups and *how* you can gradually cut these things out in preparation for your rescue.

THE *WHY*

I must confess, my family has a chocolate addiction and my mother takes the cake. Even though her hormones are now regulated, she still has cravings for it every day, keeping secret stashes of her favorite peanut M&M's and See's Candy all over the house. Even though she knows she shouldn't, it's hard to break up with sugar.

Sometimes we all can be our own worst enemy, and it's the fault of the real-life addiction that sugar has created in our bodies. A big reason for my mom's sugar cravings is her crazy, busy schedule. Although she knows which healthy foods to take to work, she still craves that energy boost to get her to the next activity quickly, whether it's her job or a tennis match.

Sugar causes the brain to release dopamine, the same neurotransmitter that spikes when someone does cocaine! Common symptoms of sugar addiction include brain fog, mental chatter, insomnia, increased appetite, depression, anxiety, cravings, and the inability to feel full. Sound familiar?

Recent studies recommend that women consume only 20 to 25 grams of sugar per day, yet the average American consumes about four times that amount! To put grams into perspective, just divide by 4 and you have the number of teaspoons—so we're looking at only 4 or 5 teaspoons of sugar per day as the recommended maximum. Just for comparison, an average 12-ounce can of soda contains around 39 grams of sugar. And this is total sugar consumption we're talking about, not just added sugars. Remember that your daily serving of fruits contains sugar (or fructose), too, so keep track of those numbers in your food journal.

Even though both glucose and fructose are sugars, they have entirely different effects on the body. Glucose can be metabolized in our cells, but fructose must be filtered through the liver. This is why it is so important to avoid that extra fructose, even if much of it is found in healthier options like fruits and vegetables. Eating an entire bag of grapes does give you some vital nutrients, and it is definitely better than a candy bar, but be aware of how much fructose is in those two choices.

Cutting back on sugar can be difficult, as one of the most common ways to "feed" stress is with sugar—so of course we crave sugar in just about every situation. Excess sugar stresses your body by causing major inflammation, taxing your liver, and damaging your arteries. It wreaks havoc on your immune system, creates fatigue, causes bloating, and is the number-one food choice of cancer. It can lead to diseases like metabolic syndrome, fatty liver syndrome, diabetes, heart disease, and Alzheimer's. And it is so very addictive, which food companies take advantage of.

Breaking up with sugar will help your body to reset its insulin and estrogen levels. Even if it's only for five days, your body will begin to slowly get used to life without the sugar highs it's accustomed to. Eventually your taste buds will reset and foods will begin to taste overly sweet to you, which makes resisting cravings a lot easier. The weight will most likely begin to drop off if you have been consuming large amounts of added sugar in your diet, unknowingly or not. Suddenly, a piece of fruit will become incredibly appealing because it has just the right amount of sugar along with fiber, enzymes, and critical antioxidants that your body needs.

THE *HOW*

Breakfast Makeover

Eating a sugary breakfast is pretty much guaranteed to set you up for cravings later that day. Since a typical American breakfast consists of juice, a sweet cereal, or white toast/bagel with jelly, plus a hot coffee or tea with added sugar, we set ourselves up for a huge insulin spike to manage all that sugar, followed by a plummeting crash leaving us craving more. Even worse, as soon as our brain realizes that it hasn't received the nutrients that it needs, it sends signals to our body to eat again, which is why we crave that mid-morning sugary fix.

This used to be me. My go-to breakfast was a KIND bar that just happened to pair perfectly with my enormous iced coffee. It also set the tone for the day, which made it so much easier for me to continue to reach for sugar. When I finally realized what was happening, I switched to real food and pumped up the protein in my breakfast. Protein added to every meal will help you curb those cravings, sustain your satiety, and keep you from grabbing that sweet snack before lunch. Assess your current breakfast plan and replace it with whole-food options packed with protein. Take a look at the following options for amazing suggestions. And do a pantry clean-out to get rid of those sugary breakfast options to resist temptation.

Eat a Savory Breakfast

I'm a big fan of savory breakfasts. You'll get the proteins and veggies you need without causing insulin spikes. Green smoothies are my go-to for when I'm on the run, but they are also satisfying when you're at home, since you can sip them and be mindful of how delicious each mouthful is. If I'm still hungry after my green smoothie, I'll scramble two eggs with spinach and add a couple slices of avocado. This protein-packed punch always keeps me going till lunch, with no need for a snack.

Prep ahead of time and have healthy options available for yourself so that breakfast doesn't become a chore. Make this a healthy part of your morning routine so that you can keep the sugar demons at bay. There's no rule that says you have to eat "breakfast foods" for breakfast. If you feel like having a salad or some meat for breakfast, have it!

Drink Green Smoothies

My smoothies only contain unsweetened almond milk, avocado, and fruit and vegetable juices, so they have no added sugar. I use a protein powder made from a vegetable source to avoid the more commonly used whey powder, which may cause gastrointestinal issues. The smoothies take only 5 to 10 minutes to make and can easily become a to-go option for your busy lifestyle. You can even pre-portion your frozen add-ins for a quick "dump, blend, and go" morning option. We have a smoothie station set up at my house with our high-powered blender, protein and matcha green tea powder, essential oils, and other add-ins so we don't have to go searching for what we need each morning. Work smarter and your mornings will be a breeze! Green smoothies also make a great afternoon snack when those cravings start.

Swap Your Snacks

Do you remember the time when you proudly said "No way" to your mom's amazing cheesecake—only to devour it during a late-night raid after everyone was asleep? I do!

Rather than telling yourself no, opt for healthier substitutions from the following chart that will satisfy your cravings. The same CDC study that showed how few Americans eat veggies every day also had bad news about fruit—only 12 percent of people in this country eat the minimum daily fruit recommendation of 1½ to 2 cups every day. That's really just a small apple and a banana! Think about this when you're having a sweet craving. I can't imagine not eating a bowlful of gorgeous raspberries or blueberries when I'm in the mood and only something sweet will do. Get into the fruit habit—it's one you won't want to break.

Get creative with these swaps! If you tend to crave sweets, for example, choose naturally sweet foods like apples, beets, berries, carrots, citrus fruits, figs, squash, and yams, and spices such as cinnamon, cloves, coriander, and nutmeg. A little dark chocolate with almond butter will knock out the dessert craving while providing you with antioxidants and protein.

FOOD SUBSTITUTIONS	
FOOD TO AVOID	**REPLACE WITH**
ALCOHOL	
Beer, wine, spirits	Herbal tea (chamomile, peppermint, rooibos)
	Spritzer with a dash of Angostura bitters
	Sparkling water with a couple of raspberries
	Water infusions with lemon, orange, or cucumber
BAKED GOODS	
Cakes, cookies, pastries, pie	Honey or peanut butter on a banana, baked apples, baked peaches, pineapple, steel-cut oats
CANDY	
Chewy candy	Raisins, figs, dates
Candy pieces (M&M's, etc.)	Frozen grapes, cherries, dried cranberries, berries, pomegranate seeds
CEREAL	
Sweetened cereal	Unsweetened, whole-grain cereal; oatmeal with berries, fruit, or nuts; fruit and nut trail mix
CHEESE	
Dairy cheeses	Avocado, cashews, Brazil nuts, and roasted vegetables
	Butternut squash puree, sweet potatoes
CHOCOLATE	
Milk chocolate	Dark chocolate, individual squares
COFFEE	
Caffeinated hot coffee	Decaf coffee with cinnamon, decaf teas, matcha latte
Caffeinated iced coffee drinks	Decaf iced tea, black coffee with unsweetened almond milk

FOOD TO AVOID	REPLACE WITH
CRUNCHY/SALTY	
Chips, crackers, popcorn, pretzels	Crunchy, cut-up vegetables, air-popped popcorn
Roasted nuts	Raw nuts (almonds, hazelnuts)
	Roasted pumpkin seeds
FRIED FOODS	
French fries, fried foods, roasted nuts	Roasted sweet potato fries, roasted or steamed foods, raw nuts, chopped veggies (celery, carrots, bell pepper)
ICE CREAM/CREAMY DESSERTS	
Dairy ice cream, pudding	Sorbet, ices, fruit smoothies, Greek yogurt, chia pudding, applesauce, avocado pudding, whole fruit smoothie
POWER/PROTEIN BARS	
Packaged power/protein bars	Nuts, raisins, almond or cashew butter
SUGARY DRINKS	
Juice, soda, and vitamin waters	WATER!

Don't Succumb to Pressure

I have given up sugar on multiple occasions, sometimes around the holiday season. One year, I was at my mom's house while nearing the end of one of my ninety-day sugar fasts, determined to get to the finish line without cheating. My mom specially made my favorite peanut butter cookies—my ultimate dessert. I know she was a little heartbroken when I told her that the peanut butter cookies were not going into my mouth. I reminded her that I appreciate her amazing love and efforts, but that I just could not give in.

That particular holiday was harder than others, as I also got a lot of pressure from the family to join in on the See's Candy guessing games and to try fun holiday drinks. Even my husband, who was also on the sugar break, cheated a little in the end. Despite all the temptation and peer pressure, however, I made it through the holiday gathering without caving in and I am very proud of myself for it.

In these moments, where you are feeling peer-pressured by family and friends, explain that you really appreciate and love them, but you are being as true as possible to your self-care needs. Hopefully, they will understand and support you.

Get a Cravings Buddy

Sometimes just talking about your cravings with someone in the same situation is all you need to do to stay on track. (This is especially helpful if you have people in your life that try to sabotage your food choices.) If you know that someone is holding you accountable and cheering you on, it's much easier to stick to your goals and be successful, especially when you support her right back. The very first time I broke up with sugar for sixty days, it was with a good friend and fellow author, Dr. Lauren Clum. I don't think we would have made it through without the daily support and text messages for accountability.

Institute a House Ban on Particular Items

What I learned from my mother's sugar addiction is how important it is to not bring your trigger foods into the house. If you know your downfall is potato chips or candy corn, don't buy them! Or, buy that one little bag so you don't end up eating a lot when you just crave a little. Is it okay to have some sugar? Yes! Of course. Especially when nothing else will satisfy your craving. But it is the quantity and quality of the sugar that matters. Don't set yourself up to binge by buying the jumbo pack and thinking that you will eat only some of it.

My husband gave in to a craving the other day. He wanted an ice cream sandwich and nothing else would do. Unfortunately, the store he was in only had boxes of four. He knows one of our rules is to not bring food like that into the house, so guess who ate all four on the ride home? My sweet husband sheepishly copped to it. "But, hey," he added. "At least I didn't bring them home!" I had to laugh.

Sneaky Names for Sugar

Food manufacturers use all sorts of devious ways to disguise the fact that so much sugar is in their products. Almost 75 percent of packaged foods contain added sweeteners. Turn yourself into a "label looker" and learn to recognize the signs of hidden sugar:

- Be sure to look for grams of sugar *per serving*. Remember, you only need 4 grams per day.
- Know the difference between natural sugars and added sugars (such as fruit sugars vs. added sweeteners) and recognize that there may be no distinction between the two.
- Check the list of ingredients. Just because "sugar" isn't listed, that doesn't mean it isn't there, lurking under another name. Obviously, avoid anything with "sugar" tagged on, such as castor sugar, brown sugar, coconut sugar, invert sugar, or turbinado sugar, among many others.
- You need to be a savvy shopper to recognize that every one of these is still sugar:

Agave	Buttered	Corn
Agave nectar	syrup	sweetener
Anhydrous	Cane juice	Crystalline
dextrose	Cane juice	fructose
Barley malt	crystals	D-ribose
Barley malt	Cane syrup	Dehydrated
syrup	Caramel	cane juice
Blackstrap	Carob syrup	Dextrin
molasses	Corn syrup	Dextrose
Brown rice	Corn syrup	Diastatic
syrup	solids	malt

Ethyl maltol	Golden syrup	Panocha
Evaporated cane juice	High-fructose corn syrup (HFCS)	Refiner's syrup
Florida crystals	Honey	Rice syrup
Fructose	Lactose	Saccharose
Fruit juice	Malt syrup	Sorghum syrup
Fruit juice concentrate	Maltodextrin	Sucanat
	Maltol	Sucrose
Galactose	Maltose	Sweet sorghum
Glucose	Mannose	Syrup
Glucose solids	Maple syrup	Treacle
	Molasses	
	Muscovado	

Gluten and Processed Foods

THE *WHY*

Gluten is a protein found in wheat, barley, and rye that functions like a "glue," making dough stretchy, and breads and baked goods springy to the touch. Despite its deliciousness, it is indigestible by the human body, causing many people to build up an intolerance or sensitivity to it. Your digestive system can't process it properly, so it can cause inflammation if it gets stuck in your gut. Common symptoms of gluten sensitivity or intolerance include frequent bloating, constipation or diarrhea, headaches, joint and muscle pain, fatigue, skin rashes or acne, and autoimmune disorders that affect the thyroid and adrenal glands (that means your hormones!).

Because the molecular structures of the gluten protein, gliadin, are remarkably similar to that of the thyroid gland, the body may mistake one for the other. If your immune system attacks the gluten that leaks through the gut into the bloodstream, it also attacks the thyroid tissue whenever gluten is present. For those already dealing with hypothyroidism and other issues, this causes major problems. It can take up to six months for the body to restore itself from an inflammatory response to gluten, so the sooner you can eliminate it from your diet, the better off you will be.

Bear in mind that gluten sensitivity is not the same as gluten intolerance or allergy, which in the form of celiac disease is an incurable condition that can adversely affect growth and digestion, as the inability to process gluten blocks the body's ability to absorb nutrients from other foods, leading to painful intestinal issues and malnutrition. When people think of gluten intolerance, they typically think of celiac, but this is just one of its manifestations. An official celiac diagnosis is quite difficult, as symptoms vary and blood tests aren't always accurate. Most people who have celiac disease have a shortening of the villi in their small intestine, which hampers food absorption, and this can only be found after a biopsy. Many people with autoimmune thyroid disorders also have celiac disease, as there may be a genetic predisposition. A proper diagnosis from a specialist is a must.

Even if you aren't sure if gluten is an issue, it can't hurt to eliminate it from your diet for at least four weeks and see if you notice any changes. Then, you can gradually start to reintroduce gluten, food by food, and see if your symptoms return. I've been gluten free for two years, and I have noticed that a lot of my earlier sluggishness and digestive issues went away once I stopped eating gluten. It's worth going gluten free to see how your body functions, and then slowly reintroducing it one item at a time to see if there is a reaction, such as the kind of sluggishness I had, bloating, and/or fatigue.

Processed foods are important to eliminate from your diet, since you often don't know what's lurking in them. Even if you become the best "label looker" ever, you can't be that vigilant every time you go to the store. The easiest step to take is to just eliminate these foods and give yourself peace of mind. Think about all the artificial ingredients and chemicals that you will easily nix from your diet just by eliminating processed foods. Now, there are products on the shelf that can still be used in your diet, but stick to the Pronounceable

Five-or-Less Rule that follows so that you know what you're putting into your body. Especially if you tend to be sensitive to different foods, it's always safer to know exactly what you've eaten recently so that you can eliminate the issue rather than sending yourself on a wild-goose ingredient chase.

THE *HOW*

Choose a Whole-Food, Plant-Focused, Clean Diet

If you eat a typical American diet with a lot of grains, especially processed or packaged foods, breaking up with gluten can seem next to impossible—but it's actually quite simple. If you stick to a whole-food, plant-focused diet with clean protein, fiber, and healthy fats you will be on the right track in no time. Shopping the perimeter of the grocery store can be the easiest change to make, since that's where produce, meat, and fresh ingredients are sold. Frozen fruits and vegetables are the only exception, as freezing them keeps in their nutrients, making them a healthy option when keeping super-fresh ingredients isn't an option.

Cook Seasonally

Another great tip is to make use of your local farmers' markets to ensure you are getting the freshest and most organic options possible. Select fresh produce available from your local organic farms and incorporate those into your meal plans. There are often great recipes available from those sellers if you just ask. But, when in doubt, sauté some veggies with a grass-fed, clean protein, and voila! Instant deliciousness.

Be Label Savvy

When you begin to eliminate processed foods, you will want to examine the labels of your products to ensure you are nixing the harmful elements from your diet. You need to be vigilant at first to watch for foods made with barley, wheat, or rye, most often in processed foods like beer, candy, gravies and sauces, spice packets or seasoning mixes, soups, processed lunch meats, salad dressings, and even french fries. Just like when you're watching out for sugar, use your "label looker" training to sleuth out the details; avoiding processed foods as a rule of thumb is the easiest solution.

Follow the Pronounceable Five-or-Less Rule
If you (or a third-grader) can't pronounce the ingredients on the box or bag, put it back on the shelf. Try to stick with foods that have only five ingredients or less; or, better yet, replace them with fresh fruits and vegetables and whole grains like quinoa, brown rice, and oats to balance your vitamins and minerals.

Caffeine

THE *WHY*

I love coffee. No, I mean I really, really *love* coffee! But the caffeine in it is still chemically addictive. I relied on coffee to wake me up, to sustain me through the morning, and to be a sweet treat in the afternoon—which totally aided the demise of my hormonal balance. Despite its antioxidant and nutritional content, or how many studies say that caffeine may not be as bad as we think, we still need to watch out for other effects taking hold. Though you may think you don't have a problem either, try going a few days (or a few hours) without a sip and see how your body responds.

If you are questioning coffee's effect on your system, you may be experiencing one or more of these symptoms: feeling wired and tired, sluggish in the afternoon, insomnia, brain fog, or nervous tension. Caffeine often mimics stress in our bodies, adding to the very problem we are trying to decrease. It can also can wreak havoc on your HPA axis, triggering cortisol levels to rise and stay up for far too long. All the de-stressing you may be focusing on with a self-care routine may be counteracted by your daily dose of coffee. And, if you are already overly stressed with chronically high levels of cortisol pulsing through your veins, caffeine from coffee will only compound the effect and leave you even worse off than you already are.

But, *coffee*! It's like being told that you have to break up with the rebel boyfriend whom your parents all of a sudden found out about. You try so hard because you know it's a bad influence in your life, but you just can't help yourself. To be honest, I was so used to that little pick-me-up in the morning that I had a much easier time breaking up with sugar.

When I did manage to conquer caffeine, I realized that I don't *need* it like I thought I did. If you drink a lot of coffee and find yourself wired and tired, or you feel yourself getting anxious after drinking just a small cup, it may be time to find a new boyfriend. I recommend breaking up with it for at least thirty days and see how your body responds.

One word of warning: cold-turkeying your daily coffee habit is not a good idea, as it can leave you with headaches and feeling pretty crummy. Follow my suggestions to wean yourself off your regular coffee and switch either to decaf coffee, decaf teas, or my personal favorite, matcha green tea, which contains healthier levels of caffeine.

THE *HOW*

Take Decaf Baby Steps

If you love coffee as much as I do, don't stop drinking it all at once, as you already know this can give you bad headaches and other symptoms. It shouldn't take more than a week or two to switch from your regular coffee with decaf, until finally it's all decaf. I did this by swapping one-fourth of my regular coffee blend with decaf, and I gradually kept substituting decaf for regular until it was all decaf.

Drink Matcha Green Tea

Yes, matcha is my personal fave for coffee-swapping! It's packed with antioxidants—and when I say "packed," I mean supercharged! It is ten times more powerful than regular green tea, and sixty times more potent than spinach and other superfoods that also help to fuel your body's needs. It boosts your metabolism and burns calories naturally, helping your body to detox while lowering cholesterol and blood sugar levels. It also enhances mood and supports concentration while calming the mind and body (the opposite effect of coffee). In fact, matcha sustains my energy throughout the day because it is rich with catechins, the most potent and beneficial antioxidants you can consume. Epigallocatechin gallate (EGCG) composes more than half of the catechins in matcha, and it works in sync with caffeine to provide health benefits, such as boosting your metabolism and immune system. In addition, the amino acid L-theanine in conjunction with caffeine sustains energy and boosts brain power without side effects. Ujido is my brand of choice, and I use it on a daily basis as part of my morning ritual.

Make New Relationships

Rather than replacing or tweaking your current routine, let's talk about some new relationships that I know you're going to love. They have done wonders for my nutritional foundation, and I urge you to incorporate them into your routine.

HYDRATE!

Thirst often mimics hunger in our bodies, and we assume that we need a snack when all we need is to hydrate. To avoid this snack-craving, drink water all day long. Never leave home without a water bottle and drink a glass before each meal. Aim for 8 × 8—those eight 8-ounce glasses of water per day—or drink at least half your body weight in ounces of water every day, and more if it's very hot out or if you're sweating a lot due to exercise. Drinking this much water throughout the day helps flush out toxins, which is essential for weight loss and healthy metabolism. I keep my water bottle right by me at work so I never forget to sip all day long.

DRINK WATER INFUSIONS

If you're just not into water, it's time to introduce you to water infusions. They're like super-charged water full of flavor and zest! I love to infuse my water with fruits, herbs, vegetables, and essential oils such as Lemon, Peppermint, Lime, and Grapefruit. I usually prepare my water infusions several days in advance, so they're ready to put into a water jug or a glass water bottle to take with me on the road. These are some of my favorites:

Super Berry Antioxidant Boost Water Infusion

½ cup blueberries
½ cup blackberries
½ cup raspberries
½ cup cherries, halved and pitted
1 quart plus 2 cups distilled water

Combine the blueberries, blackberries, raspberries, cherries, and 2 cups of the water in a blender and blend until smooth, approximately 1 minute. Pour through a fine-mesh sieve into a 2-quart pitcher. Add the remaining water. Refrigerate the infusion for at least 30 minutes before serving chilled or over ice. (Note: You can also insert the ingredients without blending into an infusion pitcher, though you won't get the added nutritional benefits.)

Weight-Control Power Water Infusion

½ ruby red grapefruit, juiced
1 orange, juiced
2 Meyer lemons, 1 juiced and 1 sliced into wheels
1½ quarts distilled water
2 drops Lemon essential oil
1 drop Grapefruit essential oil

Add the juices of the grapefruit, orange, and lemons to a small bowl, then pour the juice through a fine-mesh sieve into a 2-quart pitcher. Add the sliced lemon, cover with the water, and then add the essential oils. Refrigerate for at least 30 minutes, but preferably 2 to 3 hours, before serving.

EAT SMALLER PORTIONS OF REAL FOOD

Junk food is called junk for a reason. It's full of salt, bad fats, sugar, processed flour, and chemical additives, and it has little nutritional value. You can eat a whole lot of it and not feel full, as junk food rarely has the nutrients and fiber that fill you up.

Real food, on the other hand—such as protein, healthy fats, and fiber-rich veggies—is not only more satisfying but also makes you feel like you don't *need* something sweet. If I am craving a sweet after finishing a meal, I wait for five minutes and see if I truly need to eat any more. If I do, I go back and have a small helping of the meal I made. Usually, it's a small portion, but I figure feeding my body something nutritious is better than giving it something sweet. Physically I feel full and mentally I know I don't need any more calories. Knowing what portion size fulfills your needs is key to thriving on the 14-Day Rescue Plan. Start small now so that you can gauge your meal size and really make the recipes work for you.

YOU CAN'T EAT TOO MANY VEGETABLES!

According to a study published by the Centers for Disease Control (CDC) in November 2017, only 9 percent of Americans eat the minimum daily vegetable recommendation of two to three cups every day. They don't know what they're missing!

Veggies are loaded with the enzymes, fiber, minerals, vitamins, and antioxidants that support cellular vitality; antioxidants prevent cellular damage and reverse aging. They're low in calories and high in water content, which is good for your hydration needs. Fiber fills you up, so it suppresses appetite, reduces weight, improves blood sugar and cholesterol profiles, decreases inflammation, and slows down aging.

If you're not a veggie fan, jump onto the green smoothie train. As I've said, it's the fastest and best food you can make that delivers the most nutrient-dense meal in one serving. A quart of green smoothie has between ten and fifteen servings of fruits and vegetables, and fiber, and also includes herbs, essential oils, sprouted flax seed, and a good vegan-based protein to boost your protein intake and keep you feeling full throughout the day.

Getting into the veggie habit now or discovering which veggies are your favorites will help you to select and enjoy your meals during the 14-Day Rescue Meal Plan.

EAT HEALTHY FATS

Countless clinical studies have shown that good fats like olive oil, coconut oil, avocados, nuts and seeds, and eggs reduce your risk of heart disease without causing weight gain. They are especially critical for brain function (your neurons are covered in myelin sheaths, which is fat!) and cellular function (every one of the up to 100 *trillion* cells in your body has a fat lipid membrane to protect it and your neurons). In fact, fats are the building blocks of many critical substances in the body, and they are used to manufacture your hormones. The 14-Day Rescue Meal Plan will supply these on a daily basis, but become familiar with them and start to incorporate them into your cooking now so that you know how to use them once you start the meal plan.

TAKE SUPPLEMENTS FOR AN EXTRA BOOST

Even a super-healthy, plant-based, fiber-based, organic diet isn't enough nowadays, as it is extremely difficult for any of us to eat food containing the nutrients we're looking for, particularly magnesium, vitamin D, B vitamins, co-factors, essential fatty acids, and antioxidants. I have been consistently taking supplements for over five years and have experienced more sustainable energy, improved digestion, and happy hormones as a result. When I'm not following my routine, especially when I travel, I am not as energetic and my digestion doesn't function as well. Many of the chapters in Part II list supplements that can benefit you, but discussing your needs with a trusted health-care provider will help you to select those that your body most needs.

If you consider adding one supplement, make it magnesium, since most of us are dramatically lacking in this vital nutrient. Magnesium plays a crucial role in many chemical processes in our bodies and is a vital co-factor for the enzymes responsible for glucose metabolism. A magnesium deficiency negatively affects our ability to accept insulin. Stress, certain medications, and caffeine intake are just a few of the things that can contribute to lowered magnesium levels. While you may benefit from a supplement, consuming foods rich in magnesium, such as nuts, seeds, legumes, leafy greens, and whole grains, will also help to increase your nutritional game against hormonal imbalance. Green smoothies are also a great way to increase the magnesium content of your morning.

Rituals/Self-Care Routines to Support Nutrition

BE MINDFUL OF HOW YOU EAT

Chew your food. I mean, *really* chew your food! Slow down and enjoy the flavors, the textures, the subtle deliciousness. Let your body and mind know that there is no famine and food is not scarce. This will help reset your cortisol levels so that your body properly distributes the nutrients and allows its systems to function properly. Be mindful of how you eat and discover what a difference it can make.

Also, slow down while you eat. Since we already know that our bodies are more likely to feel hungry, less likely to feel full, and always leave us craving something due to decreased estradiol, chewing slowly and savoring your food will allow time for the ghrelin to decrease and give the leptin time to send those "I'm full" messages. This will also help to lower your stress levels. When you come away from a meal or a snack feeling satisfied and full, you are less likely to have to deal with cortisol spikes later in the day—which, as you know, cause you to reach for those sugary, carb-rich comfort foods.

Begin applying this mindfulness meditation to your routine as soon as possible. This will make the delicious meals in the 14-Day Rescue Meal Plan that much more satisfying!

BREATHE THROUGH YOUR STRESS CRAVINGS

I cannot stress enough the importance of deep breathing! You may need to retrain your body to breathe deeply from the diaphragm so that your belly goes out when you exhale and sucks in when you inhale. Your body calms itself when you breathe deeply, slowing your heart rate and telling your brain that you are in control—even if you aren't.

Anytime you feel stress creeping in and the urge to snack becomes overwhelming, try taking ten deep breaths, resting in the pauses at the peak and pit of the cycle. Inhale, pause, exhale, pause, repeat.

Pillar #2—Exercise

If you don't currently have an exercise routine or ritual in place, it's time to make the change. Our bodies were not meant to be sedentary, and our early ancestors moved for survival. In today's world, we spend far too much time doing other things and neglect our bodies. Be sure that what you choose to do makes your body and soul feel happy. If you hate running, don't run. If you find yoga boring, then seek a team sport. But don't ignore the need for movement. If you have been sedentary for a while and are starting from scratch, then this is a great place to begin your journey.

Just recognize that if your definition of working out is pushing yourself as hard as you can for an hour, five or six or seven days a week, and you find that you're still tired and not seeing results, you may be overtraining and stressing your body out. It's time to reset your workout routine.

Before any new exercise regimen, it is important that you check with your health-care provider to ensure your safe participation. If you have a history of heart disease, diabetes, or any other serious health condition, or if you have been sedentary for a year or more, a sudden increase in exercise intensity may put you at a greater risk for complications, so you may need to begin at a much lower intensity and work your way up slowly.

The following suggestions will help you build an exercise routine that works for you so that you can get the most out of the 14-Day Rescue Plan. Begin by finding the activities that make you smile, because exercise doesn't have to be in a gym and it doesn't have to make you cringe when you think about it. I recommend exercising at least four days per week—two days of cardio for at least thirty to sixty minutes to get your heart rate up and two days of strength or resistance training. Then add some yoga or stretching to encourage mindfulness and meditation while you're limbering up your body. Familiarize yourself with the routines, the reps, the poses, and the positions so that you will be able to seamlessly incorporate them during your 14-Day Rescue Plan.

Cardiovascular Exercise

Do activities such as walking, jogging, cycling, aerobics—basically any activity that you enjoy that gets your heart rate up. Try a dance party, go hiking, walk your dog, go to a spin class, ride your bike, follow along with exercise or dance videos on YouTube, park at the back of the lot and take the stairs—anything is better than nothing! Here's the kicker: during the 14-Day Rescue Plan, you *limit* this type of activity to twice a week, for no more than thirty minutes per session, performed at a moderate intensity.

How do you gauge intensity? A personal trainer can help, or if you do it on your own, there are two methods. The first is to use a rating of perceived exertion (RPE) scale. On a range of 1 to 10 (1 being "not working hard at all" and 10 being "I'm pushing myself to my limit"), you should aim for an intensity of 5 to 7. If you feel exhausted and out of breath after the first ten minutes, then you may be pushing yourself too hard. The second is by checking your heart rate and using this formula: 220 minus your age. (For example, if you're forty-five, subtract that from 220 and end up with 175. This is your predicted maximum heart rate. When you exercise, you should aim to get your heart rate up to 65 to 75 percent of your predicted maximum. For a forty-five-year-old, this would be 114 to 131 beats per minute.) That sounds doable, right? Keep in mind, though, that how you feel is a better gauge of how hard you're working. Those numbers are merely a guideline.

Strength Training

Many people focus solely on cardiovascular training because they think that the more they get their heart rate up, the more calories they burn. While this is true to an extent, adding strength or resistance training to your routine has multiple benefits. Strength training uses modalities such as weights, resistance bands, and/or body weight to place a load on the muscles. Regularly doing these types of activities helps increase muscle tone, strength, and mass, which in turn helps to improve metabolism, insulin sensitivity, and bone health. I recommend two strength-training sessions per week, doing two different exercises that work all the major muscle groups. Again, a fitness professional, such as a personal trainer, can help you figure out the best exercises for you, but there are also online videos and apps. Once you have selected your exercises, do a circuit whereby you start with exercise number 1 and do 10 to 12 repetitions of that exercise. Move on to exercise 2, and so on. Completing all eight exercises equals one set. Do this circuit two or three times per session, completing two or three sets of each exercise.

Yoga and Stretching

Last, but certainly not least, incorporate yoga and stretching into your weekly routine. These activities do not raise your heart rate like cardiovascular exercise, but they help strengthen, relax, and add flexibility to your muscles, improve mental focus, and are just enough movement to stimulate blood flow, reduce stress hormones, and make you feel relaxed. Sign up for a yoga class, or start with some Sun Salutations, a series of flexion and extension postures coordinated with your inhalation and exhalation. It's not as complicated as it sounds, and you will feel so relaxed when you are done. If you don't know where to start, try an Internet search that will show you a series of poses, or download one of the many free or inexpensive yoga apps, like Yogaia or Yoga Studio, which will guide you through a series of poses and stretches. The possibilities are endless! Your yoga routines can be performed in two longer sessions per week (a thirty-minute class, for example) or break them up into smaller sections. A ten-minute yoga routine done every morning or evening is an amazing way to help manage stress.

Use an App to Help with Your Training

There are many amazing and free apps that will create interval timers for you. These are great tools that make working out foolproof, and help rid you of any excuses not to do them! My husband and I love the Tabata app, which allows us to create our favorite workout routines while we're out of town or on vacation somewhere that doesn't have a gym. We each come up with two exercises and then create a circuit of four exercises to do along with the interval timer, and we then do a total of about four or five circuits. We easily burn between 200 and 400 calories in a short period of time—and, most important, we set up our metabolisms for continued calorie burning.

Essential Oils for Exercise Support

As always, essential oils can help you during the 14-Day Rescue Plan. Finding the essential oils that work for you is part of developing your individual routine. The following is one of my favorites that has proven successful for many women who have successfully rebuilt their foundation and balanced their hormones.

Energy & Vitality Blend

Boost your body pre-exercise to open up the respiratory system and motivate the mind. This combination can be used as a personal inhaler blend, a diffuser blend, or as a rollerball blend. Citrus and Peppermint always motivate me to work a bit harder while the Frankincense urges me toward self-confidence that I can succeed in my goals and feel good about myself in the process.

For Personal Inhaler
4 drops Wild Orange essential oil
4 drops Bergamot essential oil
3 drops Peppermint essential oil
2 drops Frankincense essential oil

Add the essential oils to a personal inhaler and use prior to exercise.

For Diffuser Blend
2 drops Wild Orange essential oil
2 drops Bergamot essential oil
1 drop Peppermint essential oil
1 drop Frankincense essential oil

Add the drops to an ultrasonic diffuser and use before or during exercise.

For Rollerball Blend
8 drops Wild Orange essential oil
8 drops Bergamot essential oil
6 drops Peppermint essential oil
4 drops Frankincense essential oil
Carrier oil of choice

Add the essential oils to a 10 mL glass rollerball bottle and top off with your preferred carrier oil. Replace the rollerball top and cap, and shake gently to blend. Apply to pulse points before exercise.

Pillar #3—Stress Management

Getting your stress under control is paramount in this battle—so if you skipped Chapter 5, read it now. Take notes. Figure out a plan to help yourself thrive. If you do anything in the time leading up to your 14-Day Rescue Plan, incorporate some of these stress-busting rituals and routines into your day. It's the first step toward reclaiming your vitality and balancing those hormones. The tips in Chapter 5 can easily be incorporated into a morning or evening ritual, or anytime a need arises. Find the ones that work for you and build your own routines.

The following suggestions are recommended for everyone, so try to work these in to your preparations for the 14-Day Rescue Plan.

Morning Routine to Start Your Day

ADORN YOURSELF IN THE MORNING

How you look affects how you feel. We all know the feeling of finding that perfect dress or those jeans that just put everything into top gear. In the morning, make it a point to adorn yourself until you feel comfortable. I'm not just talking about yoga pants and a tee shirt, though that may be the comfiest outfit for you, but what makes you feel like yourself in your own skin. Apply the Superwoman Rollerball Blend, and then dress from head to toe, and smile with confidence at yourself in the mirror.

Superwoman Rollerball Blend
This is one of the most effective blends ever.
12 drops Clary Sage essential oil
10 drops Lavender essential oil
5 drops Cedarwood essential oil
5 drops Geranium essential oil
4 drops Ylang Ylang essential oil
Carrier oil of choice

Place the oils in a 10 mL rollerball and then fill to the top with the carrier oil. Replace the rollerball top and cap, and shake gently to mix. Roll the blend over your pulse points: behind the ears, ankles, wrists, and over the heart.

Take a breath, stand up, and get into the Superwoman Power stance: stand with your hips apart and hands on your waist, like Wonder Woman. Own the moment, breathe the blend in deeply. Yes, you are Superwoman!

Evening Routine to Boost Your Sleep

Even though we may argue that our bodies don't need as much sleep as they actually do, it is imperative that we allow ourselves that downtime to recharge and reset. The standard recommendation for sleep is still seven to eight hours per night for most adults, but I don't know many women who actually allow themselves that much rest time.

Good sleep will also naturally boost serotonin levels, and when your body has enough time to recharge, your cravings will not be as intense. Refer to Chapter 7 to see how essential oils and rituals can support your sleep routine. A great beginning to an evening routine can include the following suggestions.

HERBAL TEA TIME
Heat up water for your favorite herbal tea (without the added sugar!). My personal favorite is a chocolate rooibos tea.

HEALTHY SNACK PRESENTATION
Thinly slice an apple and fan out the pieces on your favorite plate. Pay attention to presentation to make this ritual a special occasion— you eat with your eyes first, and you deserve a little something special in the evening! Next, sprinkle the apples with cinnamon or your favorite spice. (Saigon cinnamon is perfectly sweet and pairs well

with apples.) You can also soak the apples in a bowl with water and a few drops of Cinnamon Bark or Cassia essential oil for a juicy, spicy alternative.

MINDFULNESS RITUAL

It's very hard to go to sleep when your mind is racing. Chapter 7 mentioned banishing your electronics before bedtime. Reading, praying, or meditating when you get into bed are all useful ways to signal your brain that it needs to move into sleep zone. Even five minutes of mindful meditation or prayer coupled with deep breathing will calm your body into a restful relaxation to allow for sleep.

Calming Nighttime Meditation/Prayer Rollerball Blend

Essential oils have traditionally been used to support healthy meditation and prayer for centuries. The Calming Nighttime Blend (see page 133) is meant to provide calm and peace to promote a restful night's sleep. The Frankincense helps you to connect spiritually and feel loved, while Clary Sage balances your inner turmoil. Used for sacred devotion, Sandalwood is often chosen for its ability to prepare the mind for connection, while Lavender provides a natural calm and quiets the mind. Finally, Wild Orange will uplift your emotions while allowing your mind and body to relax.

Pillar #4—Reducing The Toxic Burden

As discussed in Chapter 14, toxins in the beauty products you use, as well as those in our environment, can wreak havoc on your hormones. During these two preparatory weeks, try your best to be as green as possible. You can never have too much Lemon essential oil and distilled white vinegar in the house to keep it clean and smelling fresh and wonderful! Eventually, you will be able to make over your entire home, but start small and work your way there. While this doesn't have to be accomplished before the 14-Day Rescue Plan, try to implement some of the strategies in Chapter 14 to eliminate toxins from your home, especially in your beauty and personal-care products.

Pillar #5—Self-Care Rituals

In addition to the self-care suggestions in Part II, here's one more that has helped me and thousands of other women to reclaim their bodies, minds, and sense of self. Shifting your entire paradigm of food and body image can be difficult, which is why I recommend taking baby steps at first. If you aren't sure where to start, begin by incorporating the following ritual into your day, until you make it a habit for life. As you begin to notice the results, go back and start adding other rituals, and you will begin to feel your mind and body becoming sustained and supported. You will notice that the more you do for yourself, the better you will feel and the more people will respond to your positive energy. Not only will your health and wellness improve but also your overall vitality and sense of self will exponentially increase until you feel and look like a new woman.

Living with hormonal imbalance doesn't have to be your normal. Choose to change your lifestyle so that *you* become just as important as everything else you have been prioritizing.

Self-Care Is Health Care

Whether you use these tips in the morning to guide your mind and body for the day or you relax and focus at the end of the day, mindfulness rituals can become the pause in your busy schedule devoted solely to you. Take time throughout your day and focus on your health-care needs.

Begin by incorporating *gratitude journaling*. While society influences us to focus on the negative and to rant and rave about the horrors, our sense of self needs us to be able to recognize the positives in our lives. Adding five to ten minutes of *meditation* or *prayer* about what has positively influenced your life will completely change your outlook. Gain more power by writing down what you are grateful for so that you can come back and review your journaling when you are feeling less than gracious.

Gracious Blend

While doing both these activities, use the Gracious Blend in a diffuser or rollerball jar. Help yourself find the focus and pause that you need by applying the blend to pulse points and inhaling deeply at the beginning of your routine, or diffusing it.

For Diffuser
2 drops Frankincense essential oil
2 drops Tangerine essential oil
1 drop Ylang Ylang essential oil
1 drop Rosemary essential oil

For Rollerball
10 drops Frankincense essential oil
10 drops Tangerine essential oil
5 drops Ylang Ylang essential oil
5 drops Rosemary essential oil
Carrier oil of choice

Add the essential oils to a 10 mL glass rollerball bottle and top off with a carrier oil of your choice. Replace the rollerball top and cap, and shake gently to combine. Apply to pulse points at the beginning of your mindfulness ritual.

Foundational Success with Essential Oils

I was a nutrition expert well before I discovered the power of essential oils. I learned something that floored me when I was working with my patients: I can get people to use an essential oil *before* I can get them to really change their diet. In other words, essential oils will always work right away. You'll *feel* the results. You'll know!

It is my hope that this will open the door for you to believe in holistic medicine and wellness. But if you really are serious about making changes in your life to balance your hormones and improve your health, there is no magic bullet. It's not just about the oils but also about how you approach food, hydration, exercise, and stress relief. If you're only using the oils and not making any other changes in your life, you can't possibly reap all the benefits the oils are giving you! You might not even know how potent they are if you're still making all the mistakes I once did.

Be good to yourself. You deserve to reclaim your body and your health. If nothing else, the 14-Day Rescue Plan will help you develop healthy, daily practices, teach you to make smarter choices about your body, and give you a framework to support your long-term health goals.

CHAPTER 16

The 14-Day Rescue Meal Plan Basics

Before You Start

The road to success starts with preparation. Follow these guidelines so you have everything you need prior to your initial two weeks on the plan:

1. Do a pantry clean-out. Be ruthless! Get rid of anything in the house that is off the plan. Either give it to friends or donate it to your local food bank.
2. Go through the recipe list and see which of the basics, staples, and spices you have already and which ones you'll need to buy so you don't have to think about ingredients when you're getting ready to make your meals.
3. Make a detailed shopping list and buy or order what you need. For a basics shopping list, see the next section.
4. Don't go shopping when you're hungry! It's too easy to give in to snack or junk foods when your stomach is rumbling. If

there are trigger foods that you know you can't stop eating once you start, don't buy them.

5. Don't go shopping when you're pressed for time. If you're buying any packaged foods, read labels carefully. You are going to become a world-class "label looker"!

6. Purchase or create a food journal (it can simply be sheets of paper stapled together) as you'll want to start tracking how you feel after every meal. You can even start your food journal before beginning the 14-Day Rescue Plan to get an idea of which foods make you feel good, which make you bloated, and so on.

7. Have all the essential oils and essential oil supplies you are using at hand.

8. Go through the recipes in this book and make up any new blends you want to use during the 14-Day Rescue Plan.

9. If you need extra motivation, find a workout or walking partner and schedule your exercise sessions together, now. You're much less likely to cancel when you don't want to let your friend down!

10. Create a 14-day calendar and tape it to your refrigerator or somewhere visible. Cross off every day as it goes by. I know you can stick to the plan!

Basics Shopping List

Vegetables

Arugula	Cucumber	Jalapeño	Salad greens
Bell peppers	Dandelion greens	Kale	Shallot
Broccoli		Mushrooms, portobello or crimini	Spinach
Butter lettuce	Eggplant		Squash, butternut or delicata
Carrots	Fennel	Onions, red, yellow, or green	
Cauliflower	Fermented vegetables		Sweet potatoes
Celery	Garlic cloves		Zucchini

Fruit

Apples, Granny Smith	blueberries, raspberries, strawberries)	Grapefruit	Lemons
Avocados	Cherry tomatoes	Heirloom tomatoes, red, yellow, or green	Limes
Berries (blackberries,			Olives
			Pomegranate seeds

Fats and Oils

Coconut oil, cold-pressed	Olive oil, extra-virgin

Protein

Beans	Chicken breasts, boneless and skinless	Eggs, pastured, organic	Protein powder (nondairy)
Chicken, whole	Chicken, ground	Fish (cod, halibut, mahi mahi)	Quinoa
Chicken thighs, boneless and skinless	Dulse flakes	Lentils	Salmon, skin-on fillets
		Nutritional yeast	Tofu

Nuts and Seeds

Cashews	Nut or coconut-based kefir	Pumpkin seeds	Walnuts
Tahini			

Herbs

Fresh

Basil, Italian or Thai	Dill	Lemongrass	Parsley
Cilantro	Ginger, fresh	Mint	Thyme
		Oregano	

Dried

Bay leaves	Oregano	Parsley	Rosemary

Spices

Black peppercorns	Cinnamon, ground	Nutmeg, ground	Red pepper flakes
Chili powder	Cumin, ground	Onion powder	Turmeric, ground
Chinese five-spice powder	Ginger, ground	Paprika, ground	

Pantry Items

Black beans, low-sodium, canned	Coconut milk, canned	Sriracha hot sauce	Vegetable broth
Coconut aminos	Diced tomatoes, low-sodium, canned	Tomato sauce, low-sodium, canned	Vinegar, apple cider and red wine

The 14-Day Rescue Meal Plan Nutrition Basics

My 14-Day Rescue Meal Plan is designed to create lasting success. Unlike other meal plans, this program isn't going to teach you how to "diet." Instead, you focus on nutrient-dense foods that work to balance your hormones, including fresh veggies, fruit, gluten-free whole grains, lean protein sources, and healthy fats in proper proportion to promote sustainable energy throughout the day, without the risk of overeating.

There is so much to gain by following this plan. Weight loss, energy gain, insulin resetting, hormone synergy, and greater resistance to hormonal imbalances—simply by eating delicious whole foods. It's not just about following a plan, although that will certainly help in the beginning, but about learning how to make healthy choices that support your hormones. This will create the framework for understanding the principles of healthy cooking and eating so that eating habits actually change over time. The recipes in the next chapter are designed to make cooking healthy food delicious and simple, without sacrificing favorite foods and flavors.

You will also be eliminating some foods that hijack your hormones and contribute to weight gain and low energy. These hijackers are:

- Gluten
- Dairy
- Processed sugars and sugar substitutes
- Red meat
- Caffeine

If you love the results that you get from the 14-Day Rescue Plan, go ahead and follow the recipes and meal plan for another 7 days. I have personally followed this plan for 28 days and as a result have experienced more energy, focus, and improved digestion.

Track Your Food

Calculating your basal metabolic rate (BMR) will help you to determine your daily caloric needs. In addition, tracking your consumption in your food journal will help you to assess if you are really getting the nourishment you need, and will enable you to identify when those cravings pop up during the day or when you get out of control with your habits.

When hormonal surges or imbalances cause us to crave certain foods at specific times, we need to be aware. For example, do you crave a certain snack when you're about to get your period? Before I was able to break up with my cravings, I had an insatiable desire for mid-afternoon Salted Caramel & Dark Chocolate Nut KIND bars when my monthly menstrual cycle started.

From there, you begin to develop what I like to call "caloric awareness"—how many calories you need, what is in excess, and your daily nutritional patterns. Remember that all calories are not the same; one doughnut calorie does not equal one carrot calorie in terms of nutrition. Choosing healthy foods rich in fiber and nutrients will fill you up and support your body's metabolism.

Be especially careful about what you drink. My patients often tell me things like, "Well, I'm just not hungry for breakfast," but then I see in their food journals that they downed a Venti Java Chip Frappuccino, with over 800 calories of sugar and fat, nearly every day. A large order of french fries has fewer calories!

While it may seem like a chore at first, tracking your food intake can empower you to know exactly how you are fueling your body. After only a week or two, you will be able to start discerning your cravings patterns and have more caloric awareness. Then, when those snacky times come around, you can be proactive by reaching for your Grapefruit or Peppermint essential oil and inhaling to refocus and curb those cravings.

Keep a Food Journal

Your food journal will be a huge help for you to track how you feel after every meal. It's very important to do this during your 14-Day Rescue Meal Plan, and for the remainder of the month as you begin to reintroduce foods into your diet.

You'll want to specifically pay attention to your digestion, energy, mood and any inflammation/allergen reaction to what you are eating. Focus on reintroducing one food category at a time, or even a single food. Pay close attention to how you feel a couple hours after you finish your meal. Examples of foods to reintroduce are dairy, grains, corn. You may find that certain foods cause digestive discomfort, low energy, brain fog, joint pain, sleep disruption, and mood changes.

The 14-Day Hormone Rescue Meal Plan

Tips and Rules

- Eat protein at each meal. Aim for a total of 50–60 grams of protein each day (16–20 g at each of three meals). Choose your proteins from beans, lentils, quinoa, fish, free-range pastured chicken and turkey. Be sure to eat enough protein to keep you feeling full between meals.

- Eat 1 pound of vegetables each day. Aim to consume 7 servings of raw and cooked vegetables every day. The meal plan is designed to cover your vegetable recommendations.

- Eliminate sugar and sugar substitutes. Avoid these sugars: white table sugar, honey, agave, Splenda, brown sugar, molasses, and maple syrup. The only sweetener approved is stevia.

- Eat low-glycemic-index fruits (GI index of 50 or less). The fruit list includes berries, avocado, olives, apples, grapefruit, pears, lemon, kiwis. Avoid bananas, mangoes, grapes, melons, figs.

- Eat every four to six hours. The goal is to reset your insulin levels and burn fat. Avoid snacks, as they can affect your hormones and weight loss. No snacking after dinner. Late-night snacking can lead to unwanted calories and a surge in insulin. Stick to the meal plan designed to set you up for success to stave off late-night cravings.

- To satiate hunger, drink a 16-ounce glass of water with 1 tablespoon chia seeds.

CHAPTER 17

The 14-Day Rescue
Meal Plan and Recipes

The 14-Day Rescue Meal Plan provides easy-to-prepare meals for breakfast, lunch, and dinner. The recipes were created and tested by my good friend and therapeutic chef Anna V. Bohbot. She is also the coauthor of *The Dash Diet Cookbook*, *The Matcha Miracle*, and *The Low G.I. Slow Cooker*. The recipes have also been tested by me and many women who have successfully completed the 14-Day Rescue Plan. These recipes really work and will give you a framework for cooking healthy whole foods without complicated ingredients or cooking techniques. Creating a cooking-at-home lifestyle is key to a sustainable hormonal balance.

The recipes are arranged as two types: smoothies and shakes, and lunch and dinner entrees. You'll find the meal plans provide a framework with variety. The menus are designed to serve one person, so the quantities, unless otherwise noted, are *one serving*. Suggested recipes can be substituted for vegetarians, and if you have leftovers, feel free to use them for lunch or dinner the next day. Plan on having a smoothie or shake in the morning, and an entree for lunch or dinner. You can also substitute a smoothie or shake for an on-the-go complete lunch.

Day 1

Breakfast

1 cup Tulsi or green tea

Dr. Mariza's Green Energy Smoothie (page 323), with 1–2 scoops of clean vanilla protein powder (see Resources)

Lunch

Arugula and Fennel Salad with Lemon Vinaigrette (page 328–329)

4 ounces chicken breast, fish, or tofu, cooked as desired

1 cup mixed berries

1 tablespoon fermented veggie (optional, if tolerated)

Dinner

Roasted Italian-Style Vegetables on Sweet Potato Mash (page 336)

5 ounces cod or salmon fillet, cooked as desired

Day 2

Breakfast

1 cup green or Tulsi tea

Blueberry Shake (page 324), with 1–2 scoops of clean vanilla protein powder (see Resources)

Lunch

Serving of Tomato and Cucumber Salad with Tahini Dressing (page 332)

4 ounces chopped cooked chicken, ground turkey, or tofu, prepared as desired

1 medium apple, or ½ cup mixed berries

Dinner

Salmon Fillets with Lemon Roasted Broccoli (page 344)

1 cup baked sweet potato, drizzled with coconut oil

1 tablespoon fermented veggie (optional, if tolerated)

Day 3

Breakfast

1 cup green tea, or hot water with lemon

Berry Green Smoothie (page 322), with 1–2 scoops of clean
vanilla protein powder (see Resources)

Lunch

Chicken Cobb Salad with Homemade Ranch Dressing
(page 343)

½ cup mixed berries

1 tablespoon fermented veggie (optional, if tolerated)

Dinner

Broccoli and Greens Soup (page 331)

5 ounces ground turkey or baked tofu, cooked as desired

½ cup baked sweet potato, drizzled with coconut oil

Day 4

Breakfast

Golden Milk (page 326)

Matcha Latte with Almond Milk (page 325), with 1–2 scoops of
clean vanilla protein powder (see Resources)

Lunch

Veggie Frittata (page 327)

2 cups green salad with Basic Vinaigrette (page 329)

1 tablespoon fermented veggie (optional, if tolerated)

Dinner

Zesty Walnut Pesto Zoodles (page 334)

Salmon Fillets with Lemon Roasted Broccoli (page 344)

Day 5

Breakfast

Detoxifying Bone Broth (page 335)

Green Avocado Smoothie (page 322), with 1–2 scoops of clean vanilla protein powder (see Resources)

Lunch

Ground Chicken Thai Lettuce Wraps (page 338)

2 cups green salad, or Arugula and Fennel Salad with Lemon Vinaigrette (page 328)

1 tablespoon fermented veggie (optional, if tolerated)

Dinner

Asian-Style Veggie Bowl (page 339)

5 ounces boneless and skinless chicken breast, or tofu, cooked as desired

Day 6

Breakfast

Matcha Latte with Almond Milk (page 325) or Golden Milk (page 326)

Veggie Frittata (page 327)

Lunch

Chocolate Mint Chip Shake (page 324), with 1–2 scoops of clean chocolate protein powder (see Resources)

Detoxifying Bone Broth (page 335)

Dinner

Creamy Butternut Squash Soup (page 330)

2 cups green salad with Lemon Vinaigrette (page 329)

4 ounces chopped skinless and boneless chicken, cooked as desired

½ cup sliced strawberries

1 tablespoon fermented veggie (optional, if tolerated)

Day 7

Breakfast

Golden Milk (page 326)

Berry Green Smoothie (page 322), with 1–2 scoops of clean chocolate protein powder (see Resources)

Lunch

Warm Kale and Delicata Squash Salad (page 333)

5 ounces salmon fillet, cooked as desired

1 tablespoon fermented veggie (optional, if tolerated)

Dinner

Zesty Walnut Pesto Zoodles (page 334)

Creamy Butternut Squash Soup (page 330)

Day 8

Breakfast

1 cup Tulsi or green tea

Blueberry Shake (page 324), with 1–2 scoops of clean vanilla protein powder (see Resources)

Lunch

Arugula and Fennel Salad with Lemon Vinaigrette (page 328)

4 ounces chicken breast, cooked as desired, or 2 hard-boiled eggs, chopped

1 cup mixed berries

1 tablespoon fermented veggie (optional, if tolerated)

Dinner

Stuffed Portobello Mushroom Caps (page 342)

2 cups green salad, or Arugula and Fennel Salad with Lemon
Vinaigrette (page 328)

Day 9

Breakfast

Detoxifying Bone Broth (page 335)

Green Avocado Smoothie (page 322), with 1–2 scoops of clean
vanilla protein powder (see Resources)

Lunch

Double serving of Tomato and Cucumber Salad with Tahini
Dressing (page 332)

4 ounces ground turkey, cooked as desired, or baked tofu

1 medium apple, or ½ cup mixed berries

Dinner

Salmon Fillets with Lemon Roasted Broccoli (page 344)

1 cup baked sweet potato, drizzled with coconut oil

1 tablespoon fermented veggie (optional, if tolerated)

Day 10

Breakfast

1 cup Tulsi tea, or hot water with lemon

Dr. Mariza's Green Energy Smoothie (page 323), with 1–2
scoops of clean vanilla protein powder (see Resources)

Lunch

Southwest Chicken Bowl (page 340)

½ cup mixed berries

1 tablespoon fermented veggie (optional, if tolerated)

Dinner

Roasted Italian-Style Vegetables on Sweet Potato Mash
  (page 336)

2 cups green salad, or Arugula and Fennel Salad with Basic
  Vinaigrette (page 328)

10 raw almonds or cashews

Day 11

Breakfast

Golden Milk (page 326)

Chocolate Mint Chip Shake (page 324), with 1–2 scoops of clean
  chocolate protein powder (see Resources)

Lunch

Ground Chicken Thai Lettuce Wraps (page 338)

2 cups green salad with Basic Vinaigrette (page 329)

1 tablespoon fermented veggie (optional, if tolerated)

Dinner

Broccoli and Greens Soup (page 331)

5 ounces salmon fillet, cooked as desired, or baked tofu

½ cup baked sweet potato

Day 12

Breakfast

Matcha Latte with Almond Milk (page 325)

Blueberry Shake (page 324), with 1–2 scoops of clean vanilla
  protein powder (see Resources)

Lunch

Detoxifying Bone Broth (page 335)

Green Avocado Smoothie (page 322), with 1–2 scoops of clean vanilla protein powder (see Resources)

Dinner

Warm Kale and Delicata Squash Salad (page 333)

5 ounces ground turkey, cooked as desired

1 tablespoon fermented veggie (optional, if tolerated)

Day 13

Breakfast

Golden Milk (page 326)

Veggie Frittata (page 327)

Lunch

Chocolate Mint Chip Shake (page 324), with 1–2 scoops of clean chocolate protein powder (see Resources)

Detoxifying Bone Broth (page 335)

Dinner

Creamy Butternut Squash Soup (page 330)

Tomato and Cucumber Salad with Tahini Dressing (page 332)

1 tablespoon fermented veggie (optional, if tolerated)

Day 14

Breakfast

1 cup green tea or Tulsi tea with lemon

Dr. Mariza's Green Energy Smoothie (page 323), with 1–2 scoops of clean vanilla protein powder (see Resources)

Lunch

Veggie Frittata (page 327)

2 cups green salad, or Arugula and Fennel Salad with Lemon
Vinaigrette (page 328)

Dinner

Salmon Fillets with Lemon Roasted Broccoli (page 344)

1 cup baked sweet potato, drizzled with coconut oil

1 tablespoon fermented veggie (optional, if tolerated)

Recipes

SMOOTHIES AND SHAKES

Green Avocado Smoothie

MAKES 1 SERVING

2 cups chopped kale
or mixed greens
(romaine, Swiss
chard, spinach)

1 cup water

½ green apple, cored and
chopped

½ medium avocado,
chopped

1 scoop clean protein
powder (see
Resources)

1 cup ice cubes

Place the kale and water in a high-powered blender and blend on low speed. As the kale begins to break down, increase to medium speed until completely broken down and smooth. Add the remaining ingredients, and blend on medium to high speed until you achieve your desired consistency, normally about 1 minute. Serve immediately.

Berry Green Smoothie

MAKES 1 SERVING

2 cups chopped spinach
or mixed greens (kale,
romaine, Swiss chard)

1–2 cups filtered water

½ cup frozen raspberries

½ cup frozen blueberries

½ small avocado,
chopped

1 scoop clean protein
powder (see
Resources)

1 tablespoon
unsweetened almond
butter

Place the spinach and water in a high-powered blender and blend on low until the spinach begins to break down. Increase to medium speed until completely broken down and smooth. Add the berries, avocado, protein powder, and almond butter, and blend on medium to high speed until you reach your desired consistency, usually about 1 minute. Serve immediately.

Dr. Mariza's Green Energy Smoothie

MAKES 1 SERVING

2 cups filtered water

2 cups chopped organic kale or mixed greens (romaine, Swiss chard, spinach)

½ medium avocado

½ cup frozen pineapple cubes

Juice of 1 lemon

1 scoop clean protein powder (see Resources)

1½ teaspoons organic matcha green tea powder

2 tablespoons collagen powder (see Resources)

½ cup ice cubes

Combine 1 cup of the water and the greens in a high-powered blender and blend on high speed until smooth. Add the remaining water and other ingredients. Blend until smooth, about 1 minute. (This can be stored in the refrigerator for up to 24 hours.)

Blueberry Shake

2 cups chopped mixed
   greens (kale, romaine,
   Swiss chard, spinach)

1 to 1½ cups water

⅓ cup chopped carrot

½ cup frozen blueberries

1 cup cucumbers

½ tablespoon coconut oil

½ cup unsweetened
   almond milk

1 scoop vanilla clean
   protein powder (see
   Resources)

1–2 ice cubes

Add the greens and water to a high-powdered blender. Start blending on low and as greens start to break down, increase to medium speed until greens are completely broken down and smooth. Add the carrot, blueberries, cucumbers, coconut oil, almond milk, protein powder, and ice cubes, and blend well on medium to high speed until desired consistency is achieved, about 1 minute. Serve immediately.

Chocolate Mint Chip Shake

2 cups chopped spinach
   or mixed greens (kale,
   romaine, Swiss chard)

1 to 1½ cups water

1½ cups unsweetened
   almond milk or
   coconut milk

½ cup fresh mint leaves,
   or 1 drop mint extract

½ tablespoon maca
   powder (optional)

1 tablespoon cacao nibs

½ medium avocado,
   chopped

1 scoop chocolate protein
   (see Resources)

½ cup ice cubes

Add the greens and water to a high-powered blender. Start blending on low and as greens start to break down, increase to medium speed until greens are completely broken down and smooth. Add the almond milk, mint, maca, cacao nibs, avocado, protein powder, and ice cubes, and blend well on medium to high speed until desired consistency is achieved, about 1 minute. Serve immediately.

Matcha Latte with Almond Milk

MAKES 2 SERVINGS

½ cup filtered water

1 teaspoon matcha green tea powder

1½ cups unsweetened almond milk, heated

Heat the water in a small pot over medium heat to just before boiling. Place ½ teaspoon matcha into each of two mugs. Add half the hot water to each cup and whisk until frothy. Then pour half the almond milk into each mug. If you're using a milk frother, place on the latte and turn on, allowing to froth and foam until desired texture. (Or, reserve some of the hot almond milk and separately froth in a cup, then gently pour into each mug.) Enjoy immediately.

Tip: Add 2–3 drops pure liquid stevia to sweeten, if desired.

Refreshing Tulsi Iced Tea

Tulsi, or holy basil tea, helps you relax and reduces stress. It's perfect for an afternoon or evening beverage. The Tulsi and green tea combination promotes longevity, owing to its high antioxidant content.

MAKES 4 SERVINGS

5 cups filtered water

6 tablespoons organic Tulsi tea

3 tablespoons organic decaffeinated green tea

4 cups cold water

2 cups ice cubes

Bring the filtered water to a boil and steep the Tulsi and green tea for 6 to 10 minutes. Strain the tea and add the cold water. Once the tea cools down, add the ice cubes, and serve.

Tip: Enjoy this tea warm by leaving out the ice. Tulsi tea is traditionally served warm, or at room temperature. Add 2–3 drops pure liquid stevia to sweeten the iced tea.

Golden Milk (Turmeric Tea)

For a change, use bone broth (see page 335) with these ingredients for a savory tea.

MAKES 2 SERVINGS

2 cups nondairy milk (unsweetened almond or coconut milk)

1 cup filtered water

1 teaspoon ground turmeric or minced fresh turmeric

¼ teaspoon ground ginger or minced fresh ginger

½ teaspoon ground cinnamon	⅛ teaspoon ground cardamom (optional)
½ teaspoon coconut oil	3–5 drops pure liquid stevia (optional)
⅛ teaspoon black peppercorns	

Place the milk, water, turmeric, ginger, cinnamon, coconut oil, peppercorns, and cardamom in a small saucepan and whisk to combine. Bring to a low boil over medium heat. Reduce the heat and simmer for 10 minutes, or until flavors have combined. Strain through a fine-mesh strainer, and pour into mugs.

Tip: Golden milk can be made up to 5 days ahead. Store in an airtight glass jar in the refrigerator, then warm to desired temperature and serve.

LUNCH AND DINNER ENTREES

Veggie Frittata

MAKES 4 SERVINGS

2 tablespoons extra-virgin olive oil

½ cup chopped onion

1½ cups cubed zucchini

1 garlic clove, minced

½ cup broccoli florets

½ teaspoon dried oregano

1 tablespoon chopped fresh parsley, or 1 teaspoon dried

¼ teaspoon salt and pepper, plus more as needed

2 cups baby spinach

8 large eggs

½ cup unsweetened almond milk

Preheat the oven to 350°F. Coat a 9-inch baking dish with nonstick spray.

Heat a skillet over medium heat and add the olive oil. Add the onion and zucchini and cook for about 1 minute. Add the garlic and sauté a few more minutes, then add the broccoli, oregano, and parsley. After another minute, add the salt and pepper. Mix well, then turn off the heat and add the spinach.

In a large bowl, whisk together the eggs, almond milk, and additional salt and pepper.

Spread the the sautéed ingredients in the baking dish and then pour in the egg mixture. Place dish in the oven and bake for 20 to 25 minutes, or until a knife inserted in the middle comes out clean.

Arugula and Fennel Salad with Lemon Vinaigrette

This salad is lovely with the lemon vinaigrette, but an alternative is the basic vinaigrette that follows.

SERVES 4

5 cups arugula

1 large avocado, chopped

½ cup thinly sliced fennel bulb

1 cup cherry tomatoes, cut into halves

¼ cup pine nuts (optional)

Lemon Vinaigrette (recipe follows)

In a large salad bowl, combine all the ingredients except the vinaigrette. Toss well, then pour half the vinaigrette over the salad and toss again gently to combine.

Lemon Vinaigrette

MAKES 1 CUP; SERVING SIZE IS ½ TABLESPOON

¼ cup fresh lemon juice

½ cup red wine vinegar

1 tablespoon Dijon mustard

⅛ teaspoon sea salt

⅛ teaspoon freshly ground black pepper

½ cup extra-virgin olive oil

Whisk together the lemon juice, vinegar, mustard, salt, and pepper in a small bowl. Slowly drizzle in the olive oil and continue whisking until the mixture is smooth. (Store remainder in an airtight container for future use.)

Basic Vinaigrette

MAKES ¾ CUP; SERVING SIZE IS ½ TABLESPOON

¼ cup red wine vinegar or apple cider vinegar

½ cup extra-virgin olive oil

⅛ teaspoon sea salt

Freshly ground black pepper

Combine all the ingredients in a glass bowl or jar and whisk together until smooth. (Store remainder in an airtight container for future use.)

Creamy Butternut Squash Soup

MAKES 4 SERVINGS

1 large butternut squash
(2½–3 pounds)

2 tablespoons coconut oil

1 Granny Smith apple,
peeled, cored, and
chopped

1 medium yellow onion,
chopped (about
¾ cup)

2 large garlic cloves

½ teaspoon ground
cinnamon

½ teaspoon ground
ginger

¼ teaspoon ground
nutmeg

3 quarts vegetable broth

1 teaspoon sea salt, plus
more as needed

½ teaspoon freshly
ground black pepper,
plus more as needed

1 (12-ounce) can coconut
milk

¼ teaspoon red pepper
flakes (optional)

Preheat the oven to 400°F. Line a baking sheet with parchment.

Halve the squash and use a spoon to remove the seeds and strings. Place face down on the baking sheet and roast about 1 hour, or until the skin leaves an imprint when you push down on it.

Add the coconut oil to a large pot over medium heat. Add the apple and onion, and sauté for 4 to 5 minutes, or until the apple softens and the onion is slightly browned. Add the garlic and spices and sauté for an additional minute, or until fragrant.

Using a large spoon, scoop the squash pulp out of its skin and add to the pot. Add the vegetable broth and salt and pepper, and cover. Simmer over low heat for 4 to 5 minutes, until squash is warmed through. Pour in the coconut milk and then use an immersion/stick blender to puree until smooth. (Alternatively, transfer to a high-powered blender and puree, working in batches if necessary.) Season with additional salt and pepper, and pour back into pot, heat until warm, and add the red pepper flakes, if using.

Broccoli and Greens Soup

MAKES 4 SERVINGS

2 large broccoli crowns
(about 2 pounds)

3 tablespoons extra-
virgin olive oil

½ large yellow onion,
chopped (about
½ cup)

2 large garlic cloves

3 quarts vegetable broth

1 bunch dandelion greens,
trimmed and cut into
1-inch lengths

1 tablespoon fresh lemon
juice

1 teaspoon sea salt

½ teaspoon freshly
ground black pepper,
plus more as needed

1 cup pumpkin seeds

Cut the broccoli crowns into small florets, and thinly slice the stalks into rounds. Place a large pot over medium heat. Add the olive oil, then the broccoli stalks and the onion. Sauté for 4 to 5 minutes, or until the onion is browned and the broccoli is tender. Add the garlic and sauté an additional minute, or until garlic is fragrant. Add the broccoli florets and the broth. Cover and lower the heat, and simmer for about 15 minutes or until the florets are tender.

Add the dandelion greens to the pot along with the lemon juice. Simmer an additional 3 to 4 minutes, then turn the heat off. Use an immersion/stick blender to puree the soup. (Alternatively, transfer the soup to a high-powered blender and puree, working in batches if necessary.) Season the soup with salt and pepper and transfer back to the pot to keep warm.

Heat a small sauté pan over medium heat. Rough chop the pumpkin seeds and add to the pan, shaking often until the seeds are fragrant, 2 to 3 minutes.

Ladle the soup into bowls and top with some toasted pumpkin seeds, as well as additional black pepper, if desired.

Tomato and Cucumber Salad
with Tahini Dressing

The salad is meant to be chunky and light on the arugula. You are welcome to add more arugula if you like. This salad can also be enjoyed the next day, so save those leftovers!

MAKES 4 SERVINGS

½ medium red onion

1½ pounds yellow heirloom tomatoes

1½ pounds red heirloom tomatoes

1½ pounds green heirloom tomatoes

1½ pounds purple heirloom tomatoes

1 English cucumber

1 large avocado

1 bunch arugula

½ bunch fresh basil, leaves torn into small pieces

½ bunch fresh mint, leaves roughly chopped

¼ bunch fresh parsley, roughly chopped

Tahini Dressing (recipe follows)

Toasted pumpkin seeds, chopped

Use a small mandoline or chef's knife to very thinly slice the onion half into half circles. Place in a small bowl and cover with water.

Cut the heirloom tomatoes into ¼-inch-thick slices and then into quarters. Place in a large salad bowl. Cut the cucumber in half and cut the halves in half again to create quarters. Cut into ¼-inch-thick pieces and toss into the bowl with the tomatoes. Cut the avocado in half, twist to open, and remove the pit. Cut into the flesh with the tip of your knife to create squares and use a large spoon to scoop out the meat. Mix into the tomato and cucumber mixture. Toss in the arugula and herbs, and mix well. Drizzle with the tahini dressing and sprinkle with the pumpkin seeds.

Tahini Dressing

MAKES ¾ CUP; SERVING SIZE IS ½ TABLESPOON

2 tablespoons tahini

1 garlic clove

½ teaspoon sea salt

½ cup water

In a small food processor, combine all the ingredients except the water, and blend until smooth. Slowly drizzle in the water until a smooth consistency is achieved. If the consistency is too thick for your liking, feel free to whisk or blend in more water.

Warm Kale and Delicata Squash Salad

MAKES 4 SERVINGS

2 pounds delicata squash (about 3 medium)

¼ cup extra-virgin olive oil

½ teaspoon ground turmeric

¼ teaspoon ground cinnamon

½ teaspoon sea salt

Freshly ground black pepper

2 pounds dinosaur/ lacinato kale

¼ cup chopped shallots

2 tablespoons red wine vinegar

½ cup pomegranate seeds

Preheat the oven to 400°F. Line a baking sheet with parchment.

Cut the ends off the squash, then cut in half lengthwise. Use a small spoon to scoop out the seeds and stringy flesh. Use a sharp chef knife to cut each half into ¼-inch-thick half-moons. Add to a large mixing bowl, then drizzle half of the olive oil, turmeric, cinnamon, salt, and pepper and spread in a thin layer on the baking sheet. Place in the oven and roast for 12 to 15 minutes, or until browned.

Meanwhile, remove the kale stems and cut the leaves into ¼-inch-thick strips. Place in a large bowl. In a small bowl, whisk together the shallot, vinegar, and the rest of the olive oil and then drizzle over the kale. Use your hands to massage the dressing into the kale and break down the toughness of the greens.

Toss the squash into the kale, then top the salad with the pomegranate seeds and additional peppercorns. Serve warm.

Zesty Walnut Pesto Zoodles

Missing the protein? Any type of protein would pair well with this dish. The nutritional yeast is also a great-tasting vegan substitute for protein that is packed with B vitamins and minerals.

MAKES 4 SERVINGS

4 large zucchini (about 2½ pounds), ends cut off

2 tablespoons olive oil

Walnut Pesto (recipe follows)

2 tablespoons nutritional yeast

Use a spiralizer to create zucchini noodles, also known as "zoodles."

Heat a large sauté pan over medium heat. Add the oil and then the zoodles. Cook, stirring often for about 2 to 3 minutes, then add at least 1 cup of the pesto, more or less to your liking, and toss well to heat through, 2 to 3 additional minutes. Sprinkle each portion with nutritional yeast right before serving.

Walnut Pesto

MAKES ABOUT 2 CUPS

1½ cups chopped walnuts

2 tablespoons nutritional yeast

½ bunch fresh parsley (about ½ cup packed)

1 bunch fresh Italian basil, stemmed

Juice of 1 lemon

1 teaspoon lemon zest

½ cup extra-virgin olive oil

½ teaspoon sea salt

¼ teaspoon freshly ground black pepper

¼–½ cup filtered water

In a small sauté pan over medium heat, toast the walnuts, shaking the pan often until fragrant, 2 to 3 minutes. Combine the toasted nuts, nutritional yeast, herbs, lemon juice, lemon zest, olive oil, and salt and pepper in a food processor. Slowly drizzle in the water while processing until you get a slightly runny consistency.

Detoxifying Bone Broth

MAKES 6 QUARTS; SERVING SIZE IS 1 CUP

1 carcass from 4–6-pound chicken

½ pound carrots (4–5 large), roughly chopped

½ bunch celery (4–5 stalks), roughly chopped

1 large yellow onion, quartered

3 bay leaves

½ bunch fresh thyme

½ bunch fresh parsley

4 garlic cloves, unpeeled

2-inch piece fresh ginger, roughly chopped

2 tablespoons apple cider vinegar

1 tablespoon Himalayan pink salt or color-rich salt (optional)

About 2 gallons filtered water

2 teaspoons ground turmeric

Heat a large stockpot over high heat. Add a little oil and add the carcass, breast side up, and cook for 2 to 3 minutes, until lightly browned, then add the remaining ingredients except the turmeric and pour in enough water to cover the ingredients. Bring to a rolling boil, cover, and lower the heat to a simmer. Cook for 24 hours, adding the turmeric in the last hour of cooking. Strain out and discard the bones and vegetables, then pour the broth into several glass jars for storage. Sip on the broth in between meals or use in place of water for cooking quinoa.

Roasted Italian-Style Vegetables on Sweet Potato Mash

MAKES 4 SERVINGS

ROASTED VEGGIES

¼ teaspoon dried oregano

¼ teaspoon dried rosemary

½ teaspoon dried parsley

1 large (1 pound) Italian eggplant

Salt

2 large fennel bulbs

6 tablespoons extra-virgin olive oil

¼ teaspoon red pepper flakes

Freshly ground black pepper

1½ pounds zucchini (4–5 medium)

MASHED POTATOES

2 pounds sweet potatoes, peeled (2–3 medium)

1 tablespoon extra-virgin olive oil

¼ cup chopped shallots

2 garlic cloves, minced

½ teaspoon sea salt, plus more as needed

Freshly ground black pepper

Mix the dried herbs in a small bowl.

Cut the eggplant into 1-inch-thick slices, then into batons, then into squares so you have 1-by-1-inch cubes. Line a large mixing bowl with paper towels, add the eggplant to the bowl, and sprinkle with salt. Toss well and let sit for about 10 minutes. This will pull water out of the eggplant so when you roast it, it will get nice color.

Preheat the oven to 400°F. Line 2 baking sheets with parchment.

Cut the green tops off the fennel, then cut the bulbs in half. Cut out the root end and core of each by cutting into the shape of a triangle. Use your fingers to pop out the core and discard. Use a mandoline or chef knife to slice the fennel into ¼-inch-thick slices. Toss the shaved fennel with 1 tablespoon of the olive oil, the red pepper flakes, salt, and pepper, and spread in a thin layer on the baking sheet. Place in the oven and roast for 10 to 12 minutes, or until slightly browned. Remove from oven and transfer to a bowl.

Cut the ends off the zucchini, cut in half, then cut into ½-inch-thick half-moons. Place the zucchini in a bowl and season with half the dried herb mixture. Drizzle in 2 tablespoons of oil, some salt and pepper, and then spread in a thin layer on the baking sheet.

Use a clean kitchen towel to wipe the salt off the eggplant and discard the paper towels from the bowl. Drizzle the remaining 3 tablespoons olive oil over the eggplant and the remaining dried herb mixture, then toss well. Spread in a thin layer on the other baking sheet.

Place the zucchini and eggplant in the oven and roast until each is lightly browned; the eggplant will take 15 to 18 minutes and the zucchini will take 12 to 14 minutes.

While the veggies are roasting, bring a large pot of water to a boil. Cut the sweet potatoes into 1-inch cubes and boil until you can easily insert a knife into the potatoes, about 20 minutes. Drain the potatoes. Return the pot to the heat and add the olive oil, shallots, and

garlic. Sauté until tender, 2 to 3 minutes, then add the sweet potatoes, salt, and pepper. Using a potato masher, mash the potatoes to
the consistency you like.

Serve the roasted vegetables on a bed of the mashed sweet potatoes.

Ground Chicken Thai Lettuce Wraps

If there's leftover chicken mixture, serve it atop a salad or quinoa for
a quick meal on the go. And you can make this dish vegan by substituting crimini mushrooms for the ground chicken.

MAKES 4 SERVINGS

- 2 tablespoons cold-pressed organic coconut oil
- 1 medium carrot, diced (¼-inch cubes)
- 1 lemongrass stalk, peeled and minced
- 1 (1-inch) piece fresh ginger, minced
- 1 large shallot, minced
- 2 large garlic cloves, minced
- 1½ pounds ground chicken

- 1 large zucchini, diced (¼-inch cubes)
- 3 tablespoons coconut aminos
- 2 tablespoons lime juice
- ½ cup chopped fresh cilantro
- ½ cup julienned Thai basil
- 1 large head butter lettuce
- 1 jalapeño, ½ seeded and chopped, ½ sliced
- 2 limes, cut into wedges

Preheat a large sauté pan over medium to high heat. Add the coconut oil and then the carrot, and sauté for 3 to 4 minutes, until
translucent. Add the lemongrass, ginger, and shallot, and sauté for
3 to 4 minutes, or until the shallot is browned and the lemongrass
is fragrant. Add the garlic and sauté an additional minute, or until
fragrant. Add the chicken and sauté for 6 to 7 minutes, or until
browned. Add the zucchini and sauté until browned, 2 to 3 minutes

more. Stir in the coconut aminos, lime juice, half the chopped cilantro, and half the basil.

Remove the core from the lettuce by using a knife to cut the bottom at the center to separate the leaves. Wash and pat the leaves dry, and place on a platter lined with paper towels. Place the chicken mixture in a serving bowl and set out smaller bowls of the garnishes: the remaining cilantro and basil, jalapeño slices, and lime wedges. Serve family style, with everyone scooping up the chicken and veggie mixture into a lettuce cup and adding their own individual garnishes as desired.

Asian-Style Veggie Bowl

MAKES 4 SERVINGS

1 pound crimini mushrooms, quartered

1 broccoli crown, cut into small florets

1 large zucchini, cut into ¼-inch-thick half-moons

3 tablespoons coconut oil, melted

¼ teaspoon Chinese five-spice powder

¼ teaspoon ground ginger

2 medium sweet potatoes, peeled and spiralized

2 tablespoons dulse flakes

¼ cup chopped green onions

Coconut aminos (optional)

Preheat the oven to 400°F. Line a baking sheet with parchment.

In a large bowl, combine the mushrooms, broccoli florets, and zucchini and then drizzle with 2 tablespoons of the coconut oil and sprinkle on the five-spice powder and ginger. Toss well using your hands. Spread the vegetables in a thin, even layer on the baking sheet and roast for 12 to 14 minutes, or until lightly browned.

Heat a large sauté pan over medium to high heat. Add the remaining tablespoon coconut oil and add the sweet potato "noodles." Stir often and cook for about 7 minutes, or until desired consistency.

To assemble the dish, place the warm noodles in a bowl, then top with the roasted vegetables and sprinkle with the dulse flakes. Garnish with the green onions and add a dash of coconut aminos, if using. This dish can be enjoyed at room temperature or hot.

Southwest Chicken Bowl

You can make this dish vegetarian by substituting a hearty vegetable or starch such as sweet potato for the chicken.

MAKES 4 SERVINGS

2 tablespoons coconut oil

1½ pounds boneless, skinless chicken thighs

1 teaspoon paprika

½ teaspoon ground cumin

1 teaspoon sea salt

Freshly ground black pepper

2 bell peppers, cored, seeded, and cut into strips

1 medium yellow onion, ½ cut into strips, ½ diced

1 (15-ounce) can black beans, rinsed and drained

Cilantro-Lime Dressing (recipe follows)

2 tablespoons minced fresh cilantro

Preheat a large grill pan over medium to high heat. Spread 1 tablespoon of the coconut oil on a paper towel and wipe the grill pan to grease.

Season the chicken in a large bowl with the paprika, cumin, ½ teaspoon salt, and some pepper. When the grill pan is hot, add the chicken and cook up to 10 minutes, turning once. Transfer to a plate.

Add the bell pepper and onion strips to the grill pan and cook for 8 to 10 minutes, turning every 2 to 3 minutes until lightly charred.

Place the remaining tablespoon coconut oil in a large skillet over medium to high heat and add the chopped onion. Cook, stirring often, until browned, 3 to 4 minutes. Add the black beans, and remaining ½ teaspoon salt. Stir until heated through, 4 to 5 minutes.

Slice the chicken into strips. Place the bean mixture in serving bowls, top with the grilled vegetables and chicken, then drizzle with the dressing. Garnish with the cilantro.

Cilantro-Lime Dressing

MAKES ABOUT 1 CUP;
SERVING SIZE IS ½ TABLESPOON

¾ cup coconut or nut kefir

½ cup fresh cilantro

1 garlic clove

Zest and juice of 1½ limes

¼ teaspoon sea salt

Freshly ground black pepper

2 to 4 tablespoons filtered water (optional)

Place all the ingredients in a blender and blend until smooth, adding a little water to reach desired consistency.

Stuffed Portobello Mushroom Caps

MAKES 4 SERVINGS

4 large portobello mushroom caps (stems removed)

2 tablespoons coconut oil

½ cup chopped yellow onion

1 large zucchini, cut into ¼-inch cubes

4 cups fresh spinach

2 garlic cloves, minced

¼ teaspoon ground cumin

½ teaspoon chili powder

1 (15-ounce) can diced tomatoes

1 (8-ounce) can tomato sauce

1 teaspoon sea salt

1 cup cooked quinoa

Preheat the oven to 375°F.

Use a metal spoon to scoop out the gills of the mushrooms, taking care to not break the caps.

Preheat a large sauté pan over medium heat. Add the coconut oil, then the onion and zucchini. Sauté for 3 to 4 minutes, or until the onion is tender and the zucchini has taken on some color. Add the spinach, garlic, cumin, and chili powder, stirring often so the spices don't burn, about 1 minute. Add the tomatoes and tomato sauce, then season with salt. Stir in the quinoa. Cover the pan and simmer for 4 to 5 minutes, until quinoa has plumped.

Scoop about ½ cup of the vegetable mixture into each mushroom cap. Place the stuffed caps in a casserole dish, then add about ½ cup water to the bottom, around the caps, and cover with foil. Bake for 12 to 15 minutes, or until caps are tender. Enjoy with a side salad or on a bed of roasted vegetables.

Chicken Cobb Salad with Homemade Ranch Dressing

Do you have leftover roasted veggies from another meal? Throw them into this salad as an additional ingredient or to replace the chicken.

MAKES 4 SERVINGS

1 teaspoon coconut oil

1 skinless chicken breast

1 avocado, sliced

1 cup cherry tomatoes, cut into halves

2 hard-boiled eggs, peeled and sliced

½ cup thinly sliced cucumber

½ cup thinly sliced zucchini

¼ cup chopped walnuts

5 cups mixed greens

Ranch Dressing (recipe follows)

Heat a medium sauté pan over medium-high heat, then add the coconut oil and then the chicken. Cook 5 to 7 minutes per side, or until the internal temperature reaches 165°F. Remove from the heat and let cool, then slice into strips.

Place the avocado, cherry tomatoes, eggs, cucumber, zucchini, and walnuts in a large salad bowl. Add the greens, toss well, and then drizzle on the dressing.

Ranch Dressing

MAKES 1 CUP; SERVING SIZE IS ½ TABLESPOON

½ cup raw cashews

1 tablespoon fresh lemon juice (from ½ lemon)

1 large garlic clove

⅛ teaspoon onion powder

1 tablespoon roughly chopped fresh dill

| 1 tablespoon roughly chopped fresh parsley | ½ teaspoon sea salt |
| ½ tablespoon chopped fresh oregano | ½ teaspoon freshly ground black pepper, or to taste |

Soak the cashews in filtered water overnight. The next morning, drain the cashews, reserving the water, and add to a high-powdered blender. Puree, slowly pouring in the soaking water until the cashews are a paste. Transfer to a glass container and stir in the lemon juice, garlic, onion powder, herbs, salt, and pepper. Cover and shake to combine. (This can be made in advance and lasts up to 2 weeks in the refrigerator.)

Salmon Fillets with Lemon Roasted Broccoli

MAKES 4 SERVINGS

2 broccoli crowns, cut into florets	1 teaspoon sea salt, plus more as needed
4 tablespoons extra-virgin olive oil	Freshly ground black pepper
Zest and juice of 2 large lemons	12 ounces salmon fillet

Preheat the oven to 400°F. Line a baking sheet with parchment.

In a large bowl, toss the broccoli with the olive oil, lemon zest, lemon juice, ½ teaspoon salt, and the pepper. Spread in a thin layer on the baking sheet and roast for about 10 minutes, or until starting to soften.

Season the salmon with salt and pepper on both sides. Remove the baking sheet from the oven and open up a space in the middle to fit the salmon. Add the fish to the sheet, rearrange the broccoli florets around it, then place back in the oven to roast an additional 10 to 12 minutes, until the salmon is cooked through and the broccoli is lightly browned.

CHAPTER 18

Refresh and Replenish

Congratulations on completing the 14-Day Rescue Plan! You have successfully created new habits and transformed how your body functions in just two weeks! I know there were moments that were not easy. Thank goodness you had your essential oils for emotional support! Aren't they amazing when healing the body feels difficult? Take a moment and celebrate your commitment to your health and well-being. You are walking away with daily habits, rituals, and practices that will support your long-term health.

Now that you have established healing habits you are going to want to maintain them and not lose all the hard work you just completed. When it comes to refreshing your meal plan be patient and start slowly adding back the foods you removed during the 14-Day reset, such as dairy, red meat, and items with added sugars. Allow yourself seven days to refresh your diet with new foods. During this time, add back one food at a time every three to four days, and pay attention to how your body reacts, noting your body's response and your mood. Pay close attention; symptoms may not occur the first time you reintroduce a food, but they might crop up the more you eat it.

Try following what I call the "1-2-3 Rule": eat the food once and wait a day, then eat it twice the next time and wait two days, and then eat it three times and wait three days. Introduce the foods in the following order: red meats, dairy, gluten, sugar, and caffeine.

You may also find yourself wanting to continue the plan for another seven days, which is an option that will provide amazing results. The recipes are easily integrated into your everyday life, so you could extend the 14-Day Rescue indefinitely, if you chose to do so.

Five years ago, when I participated in my first 14-day hormone rescue plan, I found out that sugar and certain grains had a detrimental effect on my body. I hadn't really known this until I reintroduced them into my diet after having banned them. I also learned that I needed to stay very mindful with my diet, or I would start to gain weight again.

Use your reentry time to figure out which foods are causing adverse reactions in your body. You will be glad you did; it will set you up for success and long-term vitality, which is why you read this book. Continue to tweak your meal plan and remove what isn't serving your body, and continue to experiment with exercise, rituals, and essential-oil recipes. These daily and weekly habits will continue to support you as they have supported thousands of women.

The best part about the 14-Day Rescue is that it is meant to become a lifestyle that is capable of evolving as you change as a person. This isn't a one-stop shop; you can make this plan work for you for the remainder of your life, so as to support your body and mind through all its stages. And even more important, there is a community of followers who will help support you through these stages, including your biggest fan—me! It's okay to slip up, it's okay to stumble, it's okay to restart the plan. The 14-Day Rescue is meant to reset your body, but this book is about changing your life forever. You can and you will!

Jackie's Story

Jackie was a fifty-one-year-old event planner and avid runner. With all her children off to college, she wanted to finally start focusing on getting healthy. She came to me because she wanted to lose the ten stubborn pounds that she wasn't able to shed with her current diet and exercise program; she was frustrated that everything she tried wasn't working. She also shared that she rarely spent time taking care of herself outside of her running. Her work was her biggest focus now that she was an empty nester, and it often kept her up late, working until midnight.

Jackie's issues were weight resistance, stress, and lack of sleep at night. **My recommendations were as follows:**

- For sleep, start going to bed at 10 p.m. and use Lavender and Vetiver in her diffuser.
- Begin the 14-Day Rescue Meal Plan to reset her eating habits and support her healthy hormone changes.
- Follow a 30-minute self-care morning ritual consisting of inhaling the Morning Boost Inhaler Blend (page 106), journaling, 5-minute meditation, green smoothie, and stretching or yoga.
- Do 30-minute short-burst exercises to ramp up her metabolism and burn fat three times a week, and running two times a week.
- Supplements: a multivitamin, 300 mg magnesium glycinate, 500 mg of ashwagandha, and 2000 mg of omega-3 fatty acids to lower stress levels and increase lean body mass.

Jackie lost seven pounds on the 14-Day Rescue Plan and reported that she continued to cook many of the recipes from the plan for several months. She lost another three pounds by the end of thirty days using these recipes and self-care rituals; she was sleeping through the night; and she woke up feeling more energized than in previous months. After ninety days, she lost a total of fifteen pounds. When I asked her if she felt that the plan was sustainable, Linda said, "I am actually surprised at how easy it was to drop the weight once I focused on the right foods, exercise, and nighttime rituals. I am loving the recipes and plan to continue with this way of eating. I'm back in my skinny jeans again which is what I really wanted for myself!"

Dear Reader,

Over the course of this book, I have discussed some of the biggest hormone culprits, and I hope you have been able to identify how to support your hormones with essential oils and sustainable lifestyle changes. One of my biggest messages has been that of listening to your body. I always say that the unexpected solution to self-healing is body self-awareness.

Now that you are feeling energized, well rested, and empowered, it's my hope that you recognize how amazing you are! You have come such a long way. You can now get clarity on your purpose and make your dreams a reality.

I am thrilled to continue this journey with you and continue to provide you with support and resources. Please count on me as your guide at any point in your wellness journey. You can find me at www.drmariza.com/hormonesolution for support and continued inspiration. No matter where you live, imagine me by your side, cheering you on for your win, big and small! I am so grateful to you for committing your health, sharing your experiences with me, and allowing me to be your guide. We make a great team!

Lastly, I want to inspire you to explore things that bring joy to your life. Find wisdom, seek understanding, learn to love yourself, and honor your strength and commitment to living a beautiful life. You are a powerful, beautiful woman who deserves everything you desire.

Much love,

Dr. Mariza Snyder

Appendix A

Resources

For more inspiration, visit **www.drmariza.com/hormonesolution**, where I've provided additional resources to support your hormone and essential oil journey, and join our amazing sisterhood of courageous women, the Hormone and Essential Oil Revolution Community.

I have also listed key resources to support your journey toward hormone balance and becoming the CEO of your health with self-care rituals and essential oils.

Additional Hormone Resources
www.drmariza.com/hormonesolution (access your full library of
    book bonuses here!)

Dr. Mariza Snyder Online
www.facebook.com/drmarizasnyder
@drmariza
www.youtube.com/dr. mariza

Comprehensive Hormone Quiz
www.drmariza.com/hormonequiz

Getting Started with Essential Oils Checklist
www.drmariza.com/checklist

Recommended High-Quality Essential Oils
www.drmariza.com/essentialoils

Custom Hormone Supplements
www.drmariza.com/supplements

Hormone Testing and Trusted Laboratories
www.drmariza.com/hormonetesting
www.dutchtest.com/

Integrative and Functional Practitioners
https://www.ifm.org/find-a-practitioner/

Understand Essential Oil Basics with Dr. Mariza's 101 Essential Oil Transformation Course
www.drmariza.com/101course

Essential Oil Accessories (Diffusers, Cases, Containers, Carrier Oils)
www.oillife.com
www.aromatools.com

Personal Care and Skin Care

Environmental Working Group
http://www.ewg.org/skindeep

Campaign for Safe Cosmetics
www.safecosmetics.org

Annmarie Gianni Skincare
https://shop.annmariegianni.com

The Spa Doctor Skincare
https://store.thespadr.com

Healthy Green Cleaning

Green Cleaning Checklist
http://www.drmariza.com/greencleaning

Environmental Working Group
www.ewg.org/guides/cleaners

Healthy Food Options for Cooking at Home

Thrive Market
www.thrivemarket.com

Vital Choice Seafood
www.vitalchoice.com

Dr. Mariza's Go-To Experts
You can find many of these experts on the "Essentially You" podcast on iTunes.

Hormone Support
Jolene Brighten, ND (https://drbrighten.com/)

Nicole Jardim (https://nicolejardim.com/)

Bridgit Danner, LAC (http://www.bridgitdanner.com/)

Sara Gottfried, MD (http://www.saragottfriedmd.com/)

Alan Christianson, NMD (https://drchristianson.com/)

Nat Kringoudis, DAOM (http://www.natkringoudis.com)

Amy Medling (http://www.pcosdiva.com)

Thyroid Support
Izabella Wentz, PharmaD, FASCP (www.thyroidpharmacist.com)

Magdalena Wszelaki, CNS (www.hormonesbalance.com)

Autoimmune Support
Amy Myers, MD (https://www.amymyersmd.com)

Tom O'Bryan, DC, CCN, DACBN (http://thedr.com/)

Terry Wahls, MD (https://terrywahls.com/)

Gut Support
Vincent Pedre, MD (http://pedremd.com/)

Summer Bock, CNS (https://summerbock.com/)

David Perlmutter, MD, FACN, ABIHM (https://drperlmutter.com)

Nutrition Support
J. J. Virgin, CNS, CHFS (https://jjvirgin.com/)

Kellyann Petrucci, MS, ND (https://www.drkellyann.com/)

Melissa Kathryn, CHN (http://melissakathryn.com/)

Mark Hyman, MD (http://drhyman.com/)

Dave Asprey (https://www.bulletproof.com)

Robyn Openshaw (https://greensmoothiegirl.com/)

Emotional Support
Trudy Scott, CN (http://www.antianxietyfoodsolution.com/)

Kelly Brogan, MD (http://kellybroganmd.com/)

Emily Fletcher (https://zivameditation.com/)

Appendix B

Bibliography

Abdi, Fatemeh, Hamid Mobedi, and Nasibeth Roozbeh. 2016. "Hops for Menopausal Vasomotor Symptoms: Mechanisms of Action." *Journal of Menopausal Medicine* 22, no. 2 (Aug.): 62–64. https://doi.org/10.6118/jmm.2016.22.2.62.

Afshar, Mahnaz Keshavarz, Zahra Behboodi Moghadam, Ziba Taghizadeh, Reza Bekhradi, Ali Montazeri, and Puran Mokhtari. 2015. "Lavender Fragrance Essential Oil and the Quality of Sleep in Postpartum Women." *Iranian Red Crescent Medical Journal* 17, no. 4 (April): e25880. https://doi.org/10.5812/ircmj.17(4)2015.25880.

Agarwal, Vishnu, Priyanka Lal, and Vikas Pruthi. 2010. "Effect of Plant Oils on *Candida albicans*." *Journal of Microbiology, Immunology, and Infection* 43, no. 5 (Oct.): 447–51. https://doi.org/10.1016/s1684-1182(10)60069-2.

Agency for Toxic Substances and Disease Registry (ATSDR). 2011. "Lead." https://www.atsdr.cdc.gov/substances/toxsubstance.asp?toxid=22.

Agency for Toxic Substances and Disease Registry (ATSDR). 2003. "Public Health Statement for Atrazine." https://www.atsdr.cdc.gov/phs/phs.asp?id=336&tid=59.

Akazawa, N., Y. Choi, A. Miyaki, Y. Tanabe, J. Sugawara, R. Ajisaka, and S. Maeda. 2012. "Curcumin Ingestion and Exercise Training Improve Vascular Endothelial Function in Postmenopausal Women." *Nutrition Research* 32, no. 1 (Oct.): 795–99. https://doi.org/10.1016/j.nutres.2012.09.002.

Ali, Babar, Naser Ali Al-Wabel, Saiba Shams, Aftab Ahamad, Shah Alam Khan, and Firoz Anwar. 2015. "Essential Oils Used in Aromatherapy: A Systematic Review." *Asian Pacific Journal of Tropical Biomedicine* 5, no. 8 (Aug.): 601–11. https://doi.org/10.1016/j.apjtb.2015.05.007.

Allen, J. M., L. J. Mailing, G. M. Niemiro, R. Moore, M. D. Cook, B. A. White, H. D. Holscher, and J. A. Woods. 2017. "Exercise Alters Gut Microbiota Composition and Function in Lean and Obese Humans." *Medicine and Science in Sports and Exercise* (November). https://doi.org/10.1249/mss.0000000000001495.

Althea Press. 2015. *Essential Oils for Beginners: The Guide to Get Started with Essential Oils and Aromatherapy.* Berkeley, CA: Althea Press.

Althea Press. 2015. *Essential Oils—Natural Remedies: The Complete A–Z Reference of Essential Oils for Health and Healing.* Berkeley, CA: Althea Press.

American Psychological Association (APA). 2017. "Stress in America 2017—Coping with Change." https://www.apa.org/news/press/releases/stress/2016/coping-with-change.pdf.

Anderson, Rachel M., Andrew K. Birnie, Norah K. Koblesky, Sara A. Romig-Martin, and Jason J. Radley. 2014. "Adrenocortical Status Predicts the Degree of Age-Related Deficits in Prefrontal Structural Plasticity and Working Memory." *Journal of Neuroscience* 34, no. 25 (June): 8387–97. https://doi.org/10.1523/jneurosci.1385-14.2014.

AromaTools. 2013. *Modern Essentials, A Contemporary Guide to the Therapeutic Use of Essential Oils.* 5th ed. Orem, UT: AromaTools.

Asnaashari, Solmaz, Abbas Delazar, Bohlol Habibi, Roghayeh Vasfi, Lutfun Nahar, Sanaz Hamedeyazdan, and Satyajit D. Sarker. 2010. "Essential Oil from *Citrus aurantifolia* Prevents Ketotifen-Induced Weight-Gain in Mice." *Phytotherapy Research* 24, no. 12 (Dec.): 1893–97. https://doi.org/10.1002/ptr.3227.

Astani, Akram, Jürgen Reichling, and Paul Schnitzler. 2010. "Comparative Study on the Antiviral Activity of Selected Monoterpenes Derived from Essential Oils." *Phytotherapy Research* 24, no. 5 (May): 673–79. https://doi.org/10.1002/ptr.2955.

Atsumi, T., and K. Tonosaki. 2007. "Smelling Lavender and Rosemary Increases Free Radical Scavenging Activity and Decreases Cortisol Levels in Saliva." *Psychiatry Research* 150, no.1 (Feb.): 89–96. https://doi.org/10.1016/j.psychres.2005.12.012.

Azadi-Yazdi, M., M. Karimi-Zarchi, A. Salehi-Abargouel, H. Fallahzadeh, and A. Nadjarzadeh. 2017. "Effects of Dietary Approach to Stop Hypertension Diet on Androgens, Antioxidant Status and Body Composition in Overweight and Obese Women with Polycystic Ovary Syndrome: A Randomised Controlled Trial." *Journal of Human Nutrition and Dietetics* 30, no. 3 (June): 275–83. https://doi.org/10.1111/jhn.12433.

Ball, Derek. 2015. "Metabolic and Endocrine Response to Exercise: Sympathoadrenal Integration with Skeletal Muscle." *Journal of Endocrinology* 224, no. 2 (Feb.): R79–95. https://doi.org/10.1530/JOE-14-0408.

Barr, D. B., M. J. Silva, K. Kato, J. A. Reidy, N. A. Malek, D. Hurtz, M. Sadowski, L. L. Needham, and A. M. Calafat. 2003. "Assessing Human Exposure to Phthalates Using Monoesters and Their Oxidized Metabolites as Biomarkers." *Environmental Health Perspectives* 111, no. 9 (July): 1148–51. https://www.ncbi.nlm.nih.gov/pubmed/12842765.

Barr, L., G. Metaxas, C. A. J. Harbach, L. A. Savoy, and P. D. Darbre. (2012). "Measurements of Paraben Concentrations in Human Breast Tissue at Serial Locations Across the Breast from Axilla to Sternum." *Journal of Applied Toxicology* 32, no. 3 (Jan.): 219–32. https://doi.org/10.1002/jat.1786.

Barrett, Julia R. 2005. "Chemical Exposures: The Ugly Side of Beauty Products." *Environmental Health Perspectives* 113, no. 1 (Jan.): A24. https://www.ncbi.nlm.nih.gov/pmc/articles/PMC1253722/.

Bartalucci, A., M. Ferrucci, F. Fulceri, G. Lazzeri., P. Lenzi, L. Toti, F. R. Serpiello, A. La Torre, and M. Gesi. 2012. "High-Intensity Exercise Training Produces Morphological and Biochemical Changes in Adrenal Gland of Mice." *Histology and Histopathology* 27, no. 6 (June): 753–69. https://doi.org/10.14670/HH-27.753.

Bauld, R., and R. F. Brown. 2009. "Stress, Psychological Distress, Psychosocial Factors, Menopause Symptoms, and Physical Health in Women." *Maturitas* 62, no. 2 (Feb.): 160–65. https://doi.org/10.1016/j.maturitas.2008.12.004.

Behnia, B., M. Heinrichs, W. Bergmann, S. Jung, J. Germann, M. Schedlowski, U. Hartmann, and T. H. Kruger. 2014. "Differential Effects of Intranasal Oxytocin on Sexual Experiences and Partner Interactions in Couples." *Hormones and Behavior* 65, no. 3 (Mar): 308–18. https://doi.org/10.1016/j.yhbeh.2014.01.009.

Berk, Lee, Stanley A. Tan, William F. Fry, and William C. Eby. 1989. "Neuroendocrine and Stress Hormone Changes During Mirthful Laughter." *American Journal of the Medical Sciences* 298, no. 6 (Dec.): 390–96. https://doi.org/10.1097/00000441-198912000-00006.

Birben, Esra, Umit Murat Sahiner, Cansin Sackensen, Serpil Erzurum, and Omer Kalayci. 2012. "Oxidative Stress and Antioxidant Defense." *World Allergy Organization Journal* 5, no. 1 (Jan.): 9–19. https://doi.org/10.1097/WOX.0b013e3182439613.

Bogdanis, G. C., P. Stavrinou, I. G. Fatouros, A. Philippou, A. Chatzinikolaou, D. Draganidis, G. Ermidis, and M. Maridaki. 2013. "Short-term High-Intensity Interval Exercise Training Attenuates Oxidative Stress Responses and Improves Antioxidant Status in Healthy Humans." *Food and Chemical Toxicology* 61 (Nov.): 171–77. https://doi.org/10.1016/j.fct.2013.05.046.

Bopp, K. L., and P. Verhaeghen. 2005. "Aging and Verbal Memory Span: A Meta-Analysis." *Journals of Gerontology. Series B, Psychological Sciences and Social Sciences* 60, no. 5 (Sept.): P223–33. https://www.ncbi.nlm.nih.gov/pubmed/16131616/.

Bronaugh, R. L., R. C. Wester, D. Bucks, H. I. Maibach, and R. Sarason. 1990. "In Vivo Percutaneous Absorption of Fragrance Ingredients in Rhesus Monkeys and Humans." *Food and Chemical Toxicology* 28, no. 5: 369–73. https://doi.org/10.1016/0278- 6915(90)90111-y.

Brondino, Natascia, Simona Re, Annalisa Boldrini, Antonella Cuccomarino, Niccolò Lanati, Francesco Barale, and Pierluigi Politi. 2014. "Curcumin as a Therapeutic Agent in Dementia: A Mini Systematic Review of Human Studies." *Scientific World Journal* 2014: 174282. https://doi.org/10.1155/2014/174282.

Brooks, K., and J. Carter. 2013. "Overtraining, Exercise, and Adrenal Insufficiency." *Journal of Novel Physiotherapies* 3, no. 125 (Feb.). https://doi.org/10.4172/2165-7025.1000125.

Burdette, Joanna E., Jianghua Liu, Shao-nong Chen, Daniel S. Fabricant, Colleen E. Piersen, Eric L. Barker, John M. Pezzuto, Andrew Mesecar, Richard B. van Breemen, Norman R. Farnsworth, and Judy L. Bolton. 2003. "Black Cohosh Acts as a Mixed Competitive Ligand and Partial Agonist of the Serotonin Receptor." *Journal of Agricultural and Food Chemistry* 51, no. 19 (Sept.): 5661–70. https://doi.org/10.1021/jf034264r.

Cahill, Farrell, Mariam Shahidi, Jennifer Shea, Danny Wadden, Wayne Gulliver, Edward Randell, Sudesh Vasdev, and Guang Sun. 2013. "High Dietary Magnesium Intake Is Associated with Low Insulin Resistance in the Newfoundland Population." *PLoS One* 8, no. 3 (Mar.): e58278. https://doi.org/10.1371/journal.pone.0058278.

Cameron, J. L. 1997. "Stress and Behaviorally Induced Reproductive Dysfunction in Primates." *Seminars in Reproductive Endocrinology* 15, no. 1 (Mar.): 37–45. https://doi.org/10.1055/s-2008-1067966.

Canli, Turhan, John E. Desmond, Zuo Zhao, and John D. E. Gabrieli. 2002. "Sex Differences in the Neural Basis of Emotional Memories." *Proceedings of the National Academy of Sciences of the U.S.A.* 99, no. 16 (Aug.): 10789–94. https://doi.org/10.1073/pnas.162356599.

Centers for Disease Control and Prevention (CDC). "Cancer Clusters—Fallon Cancer Study—Organophosphates FAQs." https://www.cdc.gov/nceh/clusters/fallon/organophosfaq.htm.

Centers for Disease Control and Prevention (CDC). 2016. "Chemical Factsheet—Phthalates." https://www.cdc.gov/biomonitoring/phthalates_factsheet.html.

Centers for Disease Control and Prevention (CDC). 2017. "Lead." https://www.cdc.gov/nceh/lead/.

Centers for Disease Control and Prevention (CDC). 2015. "National Action Plan for Combating Antibiotic-Resistant Bacteria." https://www.cdc.gov/drugresistance/pdf/national_action_plan_for_combating_antibotic-resistant_bacteria.pdf.

Centers for Disease Control and Prevention (CDC). 2017. "Nutrition." https://www.cdc.gov/nutrition/index.html.

Cerf-Ducastel, B., and C. Murphy. 2003. "FMRI Brain Activation in Response to Odors Is Reduced in Primary Olfactory Areas of Elderly Subjects." *Brain Research* 986, nos. 1–2 (Oct.): 39–53. https://www.ncbi.nlm.nih.gov/pubmed/12965228.

Cerqueira, R. O., B. N. Frey, E. Leclerc, and E. Brietzke. 2017. "*Vitex agnus castus* for Premenstrual Syndrome and Premenstrual Dysphoric Disorder: A Systematic Review." *Archives of Women's Mental Health* 20, no. 6 (Dec.): 713–19. https://doi.org/10.1007/s00737-017-0791-0.

Chadwick, L. R., G. F. Pauli, and N. R. Farnsworth. 2006. "The Pharmacognosy of *Humulus lupulus L.* (hops) with an Emphasis on Estrogenic Properties." *Phytomedicine* 13, nos. 1–2 (Jan.): 119–31. https://doi.org/10.1016/j.phymed.2004.07.006.

Chandrasekhar, K., J. Kapoor, and S. Anishetty. 2012. "A Prospective, Randomized Double-Blind, Placebo-Controlled Study of Safety and Efficacy of a High-Concentration Full-Spectrum Extract of *Ashwagandha* Root in Reducing Stress and Anxiety in Adults." *Indian Journal of Psychological Medicine* 34, no. 3 (July–Sept.): 255–62. https://doi.org/10.4103/0253-7176.106022.

Chao, Ariana M., Ania M. Jastreboff, Marney A. White, Carlos M. Grilo, and Rajita Sinha. 2017. "Stress, Cortisol, and Other Appetite-Related Hormones: Prospective Prediction of 6-month Changes in Food Cravings and Weight." *Obesity* 25, no. 4 (Apr.): 713–20. https://doi.org/10.1002/oby.21790.

Chen, Miao-Chuan, Shu-Hui Fang, and Li Fang. 2015. "The Effects of Aromatherapy in Relieving Symptoms Related to Job Stress Among Nurses." *International Journal of Nursing Practice* 21, no. 1 (Feb.): 87–93. https://doi.org/10.1111/ijn.12229.

Childs, Emma, and Harriet de Wit. 2014. "Regular Exercise Is Associated with Emotional Resilience to Acute Stress in Healthy Adults." *Frontiers in Physiology* 5: 161. https://doi.org/10.3389/fphys.2014.00161.

Cho, Mi-Yeon, Eun Sil Min, Myung-Haeng Hur, and Myeong Soo Lee. 2013. "Effects of Aromatherapy on the Anxiety, Vital Signs, and Sleep Quality of Percutaneous Coronary Intervention Patients in Intensive Care Units." *Evidence-Based Complementary and Alternative Medicine* Vol. 2013: 381381. https://doi.org/10.1155/2013/381381.

Cicero, A. F., E. Bandieri, and R. Arletti. 2001. "*Lepidium meyenii* Walp. Improves Sexual Behaviour in Male Rats Independently from Its Action on Spontaneous Locomotor Activity." *Journal of Ethnopharmacology* 75, nos. 2–3 (May): 225–29. https://www.ncbi.nlm.nih.gov/pubmed/11297856.

Cicolella, André. 2006. "Glycol Ethers: A Ubiquitous Family of Toxic Chemicals: A Plea for REACH Regulation." *Annals of the New York Academy of Sciences* 1076 (Sept.): 784–89. https://doi.org/10.1196/annals.1371.049.

Ciloglu, F., I. Peker, A. Pehlivan, K. Karacabey, N. Ilhan, O. Saygin, and R. Ozmerdivenli. 2005. "Exercise Intensity and Its Effects on Thyroid Hormones." *Neuro Endocrinology Letters* 26, no. 6 (Dec.): 830–34. https://www.ncbi.nlm.nih.gov/pubmed/16380698.

Constantino, D. and C. Guaraldi. 2008. "Effectiveness and Safety of Vaginal Suppositories for the Treatment of the Vaginal Atrophy in Postmenopausal Women: An Open, Non-Controlled Clinical Trial." *European Review for Medical and Pharmacological Sciences* 12, no. 6 (Nov.–Dec.): 411–16. https://www.ncbi.nlm.nih.gov/pubmed/19146203.

Costa, Celso A. R. A., Thaís C. Cury, Bruna O. Cassettari, Regina K. Takahira, Jorge C. Flório, and Mirtes Costa. 2013. "*Citrus aurantium* L. Essential Oil Exhibits Anxiolytic-Like Activity Mediated by 5-HT(1A)-Receptors and Reduces Cholesterol After Repeated Oral Treatment." *BMC Complementary and Alternative Medicine* 13 (Feb.): 42. https://doi.org/10.1186/1472-6882-13-42.

Cox, I. M., M. J. Campbell, and D. Dowson. 1991. "Red Blood Cell Magnesium and Chronic Fatigue Syndrome." *Lancet* 337, no. 8744 (Mar.): 757–60. https://www.ncbi.nlm.nih.gov/pubmed/1672392.

Cox, K. H., A. Pipingas, and A. B. Scholey. 2015. "Investigation of the Effects of Solid Lipid Curcumin on Cognition and Mood in a Healthy Older Population." *Journal of Psychopharmacology* 29, no. 5 (May): 642–51. https://doi.org/10.1177/0269881114552744.

Cropley, M., A. P. Banks, and J. Boyle. 2015. "The Effects of *Rhodiola rosea* L. Extract on Anxiety, Stress, Cognition, and Other Mood Symptoms." *Phytotherapy Research* 29, no. 12 (Dec.): 1934–39. https://doi.org/10/1002/ptr.5486.

Cryan, J. F., and S. M. O'Mahony. 2011. "The Microbiome-Gut-Brain Axis: From Bowel to Behavior." *Neurogastroenterology and Motility* 23, no. 3 (Mar.): 187–92. https://doi.org/10.1111/j.1365-2982.2010.01664.x.

da Costa, Estrela D., W. A. da Silva, A. T. Guimarães, B. de Oliveira Mendes, A.L. da Silva Castro, I.L. da Silva Torres, and G. Malafaia. 2015. "Predictive Behaviors for Anxiety and Depression in Female Wistar Rats Subjected to Cafeteria Diet and Stress." *Physiology & Behavior* 151 (Nov.): 252–63. https://doi.org/10.1016/j.physbeh.2015.07.016.

Day, J. C., M. Koehl, V. Deroche, M. Le Moal, and S. Maccari. 1998. "Prenatal Stress Enhances Stress- and Corticotropin-Releasing Factor-Induced Stimulation of Hippocampal Acetylcholine Release in Adult Rats." *Journal of Neuroscience* 18, no. 5 (Mar.): 1886–92. https://www.ncbi.nlm.nih.gov/pubmed/9465013.

Dayawansa, Samantha, Katsumi Umeno, Hiromasa Takakura, Etsuro Hori, Eiichi Tabuchi, Yoshinao Nagashima, Hiroyuki Oosu, Yukihiro Yada, T. Suzuki, Tatketoshi Ono, and Hisao Nishijo. 2003. "Autonomic Responses During Inhalation of Natural Fragrance of Cedrol in Humans." *Autonomic Neuroscience* 108, nos. 1–2 (Oct.): 79–86. https://doi.org/10.1016/j.autneu.2003.08.002.

Dedovic, K., A. Duchesne, J. Andrews, V. Engert, and J. C. Pruessner. 2009. "The Brain and the Stress Axis: The Neural Correlates of Cortisol Regulation in Response to Stress." *Neuroimage* 47, no. 3 (Sept.): 864–71. https://doi.org/10.1016/j.neuroimage.2009.05.074.

Deeks, A. A. 2003. "Psychological Aspects of Menopause Management." *Clinical Endocrinology & Metabolism* 17, no. 1 (Mar.): 17–31. https://doi.org/10.1016/s1521-690x(02)00077-5.

Del Pup, L. 2010. "Treatment of Atrophic and Irritative Vulvovaginal Symptoms with an Anhydrous Lipogel and Its Complementary Effect with Vaginal Estrogenic Therapy: New Evidences." *Minerva Ginecologica* 62, no. 4 (Oct.): 287–91. https://www.ncbi.nlm.nih.gov/pubmed/20827246.

De Pinho, J. C., L. Aghajanova, and C. N. Herndon. 2016. "Prepubertal Gynecomastia Due to Indirect Exposure to Nonformulary Bioidentical Hormonal Replacement Therapy: A Case Report." *Journal of Reproductive Medicine* 61, nos. 1–2 (Jan.–Feb.): 73–77. https://www.ncbi.nlm.nih.gov/pubmed/26995893.

DeWall, C. Nathan, Timothy Deckman, Matthew T. Gailliot, and Brad J. Bushman. 2011. "Sweetened Blood Cools Hot Tempers: Physiological Self-Control and Aggression." *Aggressive Behavior* 37, no. 1 (Jan.–Feb.): 73–80. https://doi.org/10.1002/ab.20366.

Diamanti-Kandarakis, E., J. P. Bourguignon, L. C. Giudice, R. Hauser, G. S. Prins, A. M. Soto, R. T. Zoeller, and A. C. Gore. 2009. "Endocrine-Disrupting Chemicals: An Endocrine Society Scientific Statement." *Endocrine Reviews* 30, no. 4 (June): 293–342. https://doi.org/10.1210/er.2009-0002.

Dickerson, S. M., and A. C. Gore. 2007. "Estrogenic Environmental Endocrine-Disrupting Chemical Effects on Reproductive Neuroendocrine Function and Dysfunction Across the Life Cycle." *Reviews in Endocrine & Metabolic Disorders* 8, no. 2 (June): 143–59. https://doi.org/10.1007/s11154-007-9048-y.

Diego, M. A., N. A. Jones, T. Field, M. Hernandez-Reif, S. Schanberg, C. Kuhn, V. McAdam, R. Galamaga, and M. Galamaga. 1998. "Aromatherapy Positively Affects Mood, EEG Patterns of Alertness and Math Computations." *International Journal of Neuroscience* 96, nos. 3–4 (Dec.): 217–24. https://www.ncbi.nlm.nih.gov/pubmed/10069621.

dōTERRA Blog. 2017. "The Blog Products." https://www.doterra.com/US/en/blog-products.

dōTERRA Science Blog. 2017. "Internal Use of Essential Oils." https://www.doterra.com/US/en/blog-science-safety-physiology-internal-use-essential-oils.

dōTERRA Science Blog. 2017. "Lavender and Serotonin." https://www.doterra.com/US/en/blog-science-safety-physiology-lavender-oil-serotonin.

dōTERRA Science Blog. 2017. "Mucous Membranes and Essential Oils." https://www.doterra.com/US/en/blog-science-safety-physiology-mucous-membranes-essential-oils.

Drexler, Shira Meir, Christian J. Merz, Tanja C. Hamacher-Dang, Martin Tegenthoff, and Oliver T. Wolf. 2015. "Effects of Cortisol on Reconsolidation of Reactivated Fear Memories." *Neuropsychopharmacology* 40, no. 13 (June): 3036–43. https://doi.org/10.1038/npp.2015.160.

Ebner, Natalie C., Hayley Kamin, Vanessa Diaz, Ronald A. Cohen, and Kai MacDonald. 2014. "Hormones as 'Difference Makers' in Cognitive and Socioemotional Aging Processes." *Frontiers in Psychology* 5 (Jan.): 1595. https://doi.org/10.3389/fpsyg.2014.01595.

Ebrahim, I. O., C. M. Shapiro, A. J. Williams, and P. B. Fenwick. 2013. "Alcohol and Sleep I: Effects on Normal Sleep." *Alcoholism, Clinical and Experimental Research* 37, no. 4 (Apr.): 549–49. https://doi.org/10.1111/acer.12006.

Eby, George A., and Karen L. Eby. 2006. "Rapid Recovery from Major Depression Using Magnesium Treatment." *Medical Hypotheses* 67, no. 2: 362–70. https://doi.org/10.1016/j.mehy.2006.01.047.

Emamverdikhan, Aazam Parnan, Nahid Goldmakani, Sayyed Asajadi Tabassi, Malihe Hassanzadeh, Nooriyeh Sharifi, and Mohammad Taghi Shakeri. 2016. "A Survey of the Therapeutic Effects of Vitamin E Suppositories on Vaginal Atrophy in Postmenopausal Women." *Iranian Journal of Nursing and Midwifery Research* 21, no. 5 (Sept.–Oct.): 475–81. https://doi.org/10.4103/1735-9066.193393.

Environmental Protection Agency (EPA). 2014. "Technical Fact Sheet—Polybrominated Diphenyl Ethers (PBDEs) and Polybrominated Biphenyls (PBBs)."

https://www.epa.gov/sites/production/files/2014-03/documents/ffrrofact sheet_contaminant_perchlorate_january2014_final_0.pdf.

Environmental Protection Agency (EPA). 2017. "Why Indoor Air Quality Is Important to Schools." https://www.epa.gov/iaq-schools/why-indoor-air -quality-important-schools.

Environmental Working Group (EWG). 2005. "Body Burden: The Pollution in Newborns—A Benchmark Investigation of Industrial Chemicals, Pollutants and Pesticides in Umbilical Cord Blood." https://www.ewg.org/research/ body-burden-pollution-newborns.

Environmental Working Group (EWG). 2014. "EWG's 2014 Shopper's Guide to Avoiding GMO Food." https://www.ewg.org/research/shoppers-guide-to -avoiding-gmos.

Environmental Working Group (EWG). 2017. "EWG's 2017 Shopper's Guide to Pesticides in Produce." https://www.ewg.org/foodnews/summary.php.

Environmental Working Group (EWG). 2017. "EWG's Guide to Healthy Cleaning—Cleaning Supplies and Your Health." https://www.ewg.org/ guides/cleaners/content/cleaners_and_health.

Environmental Working Group (EWG). 2017. "Exposures Add Up—Survey Results." http://www.ewg.org/skindeep/2004/06/15/exposures-add-up -survey-results/.

Environmental Working Group (EWG). 2013. "Dirty Dozen Endocrine Disruptors—12 Hormone-Altering Chemicals and How to Avoid Them." https://www.ewg.org/research/dirty-dozen-list-endocrine-disruptors.

Environmental Working Group (EWG). 2017. "EWG's Skin Deep Cosmetics Database." http://ewg.com/skindeep.

Environmental Protection Agency (EPA). 2016. "Research on Endocrine Disruptors." https://www.epa.gov/chemical-research/research-endocrine -disruptors.

Ercal, N., H. Gurer-Orhan, and N. Aykin-Burns. 2001. "Toxic Metals and Oxidative Stress Part I: Mechanisms Involved in Metal-Induced Oxidative Damage." *Current Topics in Medicinal Chemistry* 1, no. 6 (Dec.): 529–39. https:// www.ncbi.nlm.nih.gov/pubmed/11895129.

Erk, S., M. Kiefer, J. Grothe, A. P. Wunderlich, M. Spitzer, and H. Walter. 2003. "Emotional Context Modulates Subsequent Memory Effect." *Neuroimage* 18, no. 2 (Feb.): 439–47. https://www.ncbi.nlm.nih.gov/pubmed/12595197.

Espeland, M. A., S. R. Rapp, S. A. Shumaker, R. Brunner, J. E. Manson, B. B. Sherwin, J. Hsia, K. L. Margolis, P. E. Hogan, R. Wallace, et al. 2004. "Conjugated Equine Estrogens and Global Cognitive Function in Postmenopausal Women: Women's Health Initiative Memory Study." *JAMA* 291, no. 24 (June): 2959–68. https://www.ncbi.nlm.nih.gov/pubmed/15213207/.

Fariss, Marc W., Catherine B. Chan, Manisha Patel, Bennett Van Houten, and Sten Orrenius. 2005. "Role of Mitochondria in Toxic Oxidative Stress." *Molecular Interventions* 5, no. 2 (Apr.): 94–111. https://doi.org/10.1124/mi.5.2.7.

Fatemeh, A., H. Mobedi, and N. Roozbeh. 2016. "Hops for Menopausal Vasomotor Symptoms: Mechanisms of Action." *Journal of Menopausal Medicine* 22, no. 2 (Aug.): 62–64. https://doi.org/10.6118/jmm.2016.22.2.62.

Fibler, M., and A. Quante. 2014. "A Case Series on the Use of Lavendula Oil Capsules in Patients Suffering from Major Depressive Disorder and Symptoms of Psychomotor Agitation, Insomnia and Anxiety." *Complementary Therapies in Medicine* 22, no. 1 (Feb.): 63–69. https://doi.org/10.1016/j.ctim.2013.11.008.

Field, T., M. Hernandez-Reif, M. Diego, S. Schanberg, and C. Kuhn. 2005. "Cortisol Decreases and Serotonin and Dopamine Increase Following Massage Therapy." *International Journal of Neuroscience* 115, no. 10 (Nov.): 1397–413. https://www.ncbi.nlm.nih.gov/pubmed/16162447.

Forrest, K. Y., and W. L. Stuhldreher. 2011. "Prevalence and Correlates of Vitamin D Deficiency in US Adults." *Nutrition Research* 31, no. 1 (Jan): 48–54. https://doi.org/10.1016/j.nutres.2010.12.001.

Fowler, P. A., M. Bellingham, K. D. Sinclair, N. P. Evans, P. Pocar, B. Fischer, K. Schaedlich, J. S. Schmidt, M. R. Amezaga, S. Bhattacharya, et al. 2012. "Impact of Endocrine-Disrupting Compounds (EDCs) on Female Reproductive Health." *Molecular and Cellular Endocrinology* 355, no. 2 (May): 231–39. https://doi.org/10.1016/j.mce.2011.10.021.

Fukumoto, Syuichi, Aya Morishita, Kohei Furutachi, Takehiko Terashima, Tsutomu Nakayama, and Hidehiko Yokogoshi. 2008. "Effect of Flavour Components in Lemon Essential Oil on Physical or Psychological Stress." *Stress Health* 24, no. 1 (Oct.): 3–12. https://doi.org/10.1002/smi.1158.

Garabadu, Debapriya, Ankit Shah, Sanjay Singh, and Sairam Krishnamurthy. 2015. "Protective Effect of Eugenol Against Restraint Stress-Induced Gastrointestinal Dysfunction: Potential Use in Irritable Bowel Syndrome." *Pharmaceutical Biology* 53, no. 7 (July): 968–74. https://doi.org/10.3109/13880209.2014.950674.

Geller, S. E. and L. Studee. 2005. "Botanical and Dietary Supplements for Menopausal Symptoms: What Works, What Doesn't." *Journal of Women's Health (Larchmt)* 14, no. 7 (Sept.): 634–49. https://doi.org/10.10089/jwh.2005.14.634.

Gershon, M. D. 1999. "The Enteric Nervous System: A Second Brain." *Hospital Practice* 34, no. 7 (July): 31–32, 35–38, 41–42. https://www.ncbi.nlm.nih.gov/pubmed/10418549.

Gershon, M. D. 1999. *The Second Brain—A Groundbreaking New Understanding of Nervous Disorders of the Stomach and Intestine.* New York: Harper Perennial.

Ghelardini, Carla, Nicoletta Galeotti, Giuseppe Salvatore, and Gabriela Mazzanti. 1999. "Local Anaesthetic Activity of the Essential Oil of *Lavandula angustifolia*." *Planta Medica* 65, no. 8 (Dec.): 700–703. https://doi.org/10.1055/s-1999-14045.

Gibbs, D. M. 1986. "Vasopressin and Oxytocin: Hypothalamic Modulators of the Stress Response: A Review." *Psychoneuroendocrinology* 11, no. 2: 131–39. https://www.ncbi.nlm.nih.gov/pubmed/3018820.

Gillerman, Hope. 2016. *Essential Oils Every Day.* New York: HarperElixir.

Goel, Namni, Hyungsoo Kim, and Raymund P. Lao. 2005. "An Olfactory Stimulus Modifies Nighttime Sleep in Young Men and Women." *Chronobiology International* 22, no. 5 (July): 889–904. https://doi.org/10.1080/07420520500263276.

Gottfried, Sara. 2013. *The Hormone Cure*. New York: Scribner.

Graziottin, A. 2000. "Libido: The Biologic Scenario." *Maturitas* 34 Suppl. 1(Jan.): S9–16. https://www.ncbi.nlm.nih.gov/pubmed/10759059.

Gray, J. R., T. S. Braver, and M. E. Raichle. 2002. "Integration of Emotion and Cognition in the Lateral Prefrontal Cortex." *Proceedings of the National Academy Sciences of the U.S.A.* 99, no. 6 (Mar.): 4115–20. http://doi.org/10.1073/pnas.062381899.

Group, Dr. Edward. 2015. "3 Ways Endocrine Disruptors Destroy Your Health." *Global Healing Center.* http://globalhealingcenter.com/natural-health/3-ways-endocrine-disruptors-destroy-health.

Gupta, Subash C., Sahdeo Prasad, Ji Hye Kim, Sridevi Patchva, Lauren J. Webb, Indira K. Priyadarsini, and Bharat B. Aggarwai. 2011. "Multitargeting by Curcumin as Revealed by Molecular Interaction Studies." *Natural Product Reports* 28, no. 12 (Nov.): 1937–55. https://doi.org/10.1039/c1np00051a.

Guzmán, Y. F., N. C. Tronson, V. Jovasevic, K. Sato, A. L. Guedea, H. Mizukami, K. Nishimori, and J. Radulovic. 2013. "Fear-enhancing Effects of Septal Oxytocin Receptors." *Nature Neuroscience* 16, no. 9 (Sept.): 1185–87. https://doi.org/10.1038/nn.3465.

Habtemariam, S. 2016. "The Therapeutic Potential of Rosemary (*Rosmarinus officialis*) Diterpenes for Alzheimer's Disease." *Evidence-Based Complementary and Alternative Medicine* Vol. 2016: 2680409. https://doi.org/10.1155/2016/2680409.

Hackney, A. C., A. Kallman, K. P. Hosick, D. A. Rubin, and C. L. Battaglini. 2012. "Thyroid Hormonal Responses to Intensive Interval versus Steady-State Endurance Exercise Sessions." *Hormones* (Athens) 11, no. 1 (Jan.–Mar.): 54–60. https://www.ncbi.nlm.nih.gov/pubmed/22450344.

Hadhazy, Adam. 2010. "Think Twice: How the Gut's 'Second Brain' Influences Mood and Well-Being." *Scientific American* (Feb). https://www.scientificamerican.com/article/gut-second-brain/.

Hamann, S. 2001. "Cognitive and Neural Mechanisms of Emotional Memory." *Trends in Cognitive Sciences* 5, no. 9 (Sept.): 394–400. https://www.ncbi.nlm.nih.gov/pubmed/11520704.

Hao, Y., A. Shabanpoor, and G. A. Metz. 2017. "Stress and Corticosterone Alter Synaptic Plasticity in a Rat Model of Parkinson's Disease." *Neuroscience Letters* 651 (June): 79–87. https://doi.org/10.1016/j.neulet.2017.04.063.

Hare, Brendan D., Jacob A. Beierle, Donna J. Toufexis, Sayamwong E. Hammack, and William A. Falls. 2014. "Exercise-associated Changes in the Corticosterone Response to Acute Restraint Stress: Evidence for Increased Adrenal Sensitivity and Reduced Corticosterone Response Duration." *Neuropsychopharmacology* 39, no. 5 (Apr.): 1262–69. https://doi.org/10.1038/npp.2013.329.

Harman, S. M. 2014. "Menopausal Hormone Treatment Cardiovascular Disease: Another Look at an Unresolved Conundrum." *Fertility and Sterility* 101, no. 4 (Apr.): 887–97. https://doi.org/10.1016/j.fertnstert.2014.02.042.

Hartling, L., A. S. Newton, Y. Liang, H. Jou, K. Hewson, T. P. Kiassen, and S. Curtis. 2013. "Music to Reduce Pain and Distress in the Pediatric Emergency Department." *JAMA Pediatrics* 167, no. 9 (Sept.): 826–35. https://doi.org/10.1001/jamapediatrics.2013.200.

Hasselmo, M. E. 2006. "The Role of Acetylcholine in Learning and Memory." *Current Opinion in Neurobiology* 16, no. 6 (Dec.): 710–15. https://doi.org/10.1016/j.conb.2006.09.002.

Hein, A., F. C. Thiel, C. M. Bayer, P. A. Fasching, L. Häberle, M. P. Lux, S. P. Renner, S. M. Jud, M. G. Schrauder, A. Müller, et al. 2013. "Hormone Replacement Therapy and Prognosis in Ovarian Cancer Patients." *European Journal of Cancer Prevention* 22, no. 1 (Jan.): 52–58. https://doi.org/10.1097/CEJ.0b013e328355ec22.

Heiss, G., R. Wallace, G. L. Anderson, A. Aragaki, S. A. Beresford, R. Brzyski, R. T. Chlebowski, M. Gass, A. LaCroix, J. E. Manson, et al. 2008. "Health Risks and Benefits 3 Years After Stopping Randomized Treatment with Estrogen and Progestin." *JAMA* 299, no. 9 (Mar.): 1036–45. https://doi.org/10.1001/jama.299.9.1036.

Herro, E., and S. E. Jacob. 2010. "*Mentha piperita* (Peppermint)." *Dermatitis* 21, no. 6 (Nov.–Dec.): 327–29. https://www.ncbi.nlm.nih.gov/pubmed/21144345.

Heyerick, Arne, Stefaan M. Vervarcke, Herman Depypere, and Denis De Keukeleire. 2006. "A First Prospective, Randomized, Double-Blind, Placebo-Controlled Study on the Use of a Standardized Hop Extract to Alleviate Menopausal Discomforts." *Maturitas* 54, no. 2 (May): 164–75. https://doi.org/10.1016/j.maturitas.2005.10.005.

Hill, Dr. David. 2015. "The Power of Aroma." *DōTERRA Living Magazine.* https://www.doterra.com/US/en/brochures-magazines-doterra-living-spring-2015-the-power-of-aroma.

Hirsch, A. R., M.D., and R. Gomez. 1995. "Weight Reduction Through Inhalation of Odorants." *Journal of Neurological and Orthopedic Medicine and Surgery* 16: 26–31.

Hirshkowitz, Max, Kaitlyn Whiton, Steven M. Albert, Cathy Alessi, Oliviero Bruni, Lydia DonCarlos, Nancy Hazen, John Herman, Eliot S. Katz, Leila Kheirandish-Gozal, et al. 2015. "National Sleep Foundation's Sleep Time Duration Recommendations: Methodology and Results Summary." *Sleep Health—Journal of the National Sleep Foundation* 1, no. 1 (Mar.): 40–43. https://doi.org/10.1016/j.sleh.2014.12.010.

Hongratanaworakit, T., and G. Buchbauer. 2006. "Relaxing Effect of Ylang Ylang Oil on Humans After Transdermal Absorption." *Phytotherapy Research* 20, no. 9: 758–63. https://doi.org/10.1002/ptr.1950.

Hormann, Annette M., Frederick S. vom Saal, Susan C. Nagel, Richard W. Stahlhut, Carol L. Moyer, Mark R. Ellersieck, Wade V. Welshons, Pierre-Louis Toutain, and Julia A. Taylor. 2014. "Holding Thermal Receipt Paper and Eating Food After Using Hand Sanitizer Results in High Serum Bioactive and Urine Total Levels of Bisphenol A (BPA)." *PLoS One* 9, no. 10 (Oct.): e110509. https://doi.org/10.1371/journal.pone.0110509.

Hou, Ningqi, Susan Hong, Wenli Wang, Olufunmilayo I. Olopade, James J. Dignam, and Dezheng Huo. 2013. "Hormone Replacement Therapy and Breast Cancer: Heterogeneous Risks by Race, Weight, and Breast Density." *Journal of the National Cancer Institute* 105, no. 18 (Sept.): 1365–72. https://doi.org/10.1093/jnci/djt207.

Hu, C., and D. D. Kitts. 2003. "Antioxidant, Prooxidant, and Cytotoxic Activities of Solvent-Fractionated Dandelion (*Taraxacum officinale*) Flower Extracts In Vitro." *Journal of Agricultural and Food Chemistry* 51, no. 1 (Jan.): 301–10. https://doi.org/10.1021/jf0258858.

Hucklenbroich, Joerg, Rebecca Klein, Bernd Neumaier, Rudolf Graf, Gereon Rudolf Fink, Michael Schroeter, and Maria Adele Rueger. 2014. "Aromatic-Turmerone Induces Neural Stem Cell Proliferation In Vitro and In Vivo." *Stem Cell Research & Therapy* 5, no 4. (Sept.): 100. https://doi.org/10.1186/scrt500.

Hur, Myung-Haeng, Myeong Soo Lee, Ka-Yeon Seong, and Mi-Kyoung Lee. 2012. "Aromatherapy Massage on the Abdomen for Alleviating Menstrual Pain in High School Girls: A Preliminary Controlled Clinical Study." *Evidence-Based Complementary and Alternative Medicine* Vol. 2012: 187163. https://doi.org/10.1155/2012/187163.

Hwang, J. H. 2006. "The Effects of the Inhalation Method Using Essential Oils on Blood Pressure and Stress Responses of Clients with Essential Hypertension." *Taehan Kanho Hakhoe Chi* 36, no. 7 (Dec.): 1123–34. https://www.ncbi.nlm.nih.gov/pubmed/17211115.

Ishaque, Sana, Larissa Shamseer, Cecilia Bukutu, and Sunita Vohra. 2012. "*Rhodiola rosea* for Physical and Mental Fatigue: A Systematic Review." *BMC Complementary & Alternative Medicine* 12: 70. https://doi.org/10.1186/1472-6882-12-70.

Jenkins, T. A., J. C. Nguyen, K. E. Polglaze, and P. P. Bertrand. 2016. "Influence of Tryptophan and Serotonin on Mood and Cognition with a Possible Role of the Gut-Brain Axis." *Nutrients* 8, no. 1 (Jan.): 56. https://doi.org/10.3390/nu8010056.

Jones, Emma K., Janelle R. Jurgenson, Judith M. Katzenellenbogen, and Sandra C. Thompson. 2012. "Menopause and the Influence of Culture: Another Gap for Indigenous Australian Women?" *BMC Women's Health* 12: 43. https://doi.org/10.1186/1472-6874-12-43.

Kaaks, R. 1996. "Nutrition, Hormones, and Breast Cancer: Is Insulin the Missing Link?" *Cancer Causes & Control* 7, no. 6 (Nov.): 605–25. https://link.springer.com/article/10.1007/BF00051703.

Kalleinen, N., P. Polo-Kantola, K. Irjala, T. Porkka-Heiskanen, T. Vahlberg, A. Virkki, and O. Polo. 2008. "24-hour Serum Levels of Growth Hormone, Prolactin, and Cortisol in Pre- and Postmenopausal Women: The Effect of

Combined Estrogen and Progestin Treatment." *Journal of Clinical Endocrinology & Metabolism* 93, no. 5 (May): 1655–61. https://doi.org/10.1210/jc.2007-2677.

Kaluzna-Czaplińska, J., P. Gatarek, S. Chirumbolo, M. S. Chartrand, and G. Bjørklund. 2017. "How Important Is Tryptophan in Human Health?" *Critical Reviews in Food Science and Nutrition* (Aug.): 1–17. https://doi.org/10.1080/10408398.2017.1357534.

Karama, S., S. Ducharme, J. Corley, F. Chouinard-Decorte, J. M. Starr, J. M. Wardlaw, M. E. Bastin, and I. J. Deary. 2015. "Cigarette Smoking and Thinning of the Brain's Cortex." *Molecular Psychiatry* 20, no. 6 (June): 778–85. https://doi.org/10.1038/mp.2014.187.

Katan, M., Y. P. Moon, M. C. Paik, R. L. Sacco, C. B. Wright, and M. S. Elkind. 2013. "Infections Burden and Cognitive Function: The Northern Manhattan Study." *Neurology* 80, no. 13 (Mar.): 1209–15. https://doi.org/10.1212/WNL.0b013e3182896e79.

Kato-Kataoka, Akito, Kensei Nishida, Mai Takada, Mitsuhisa Kawai, Hiroko Kikuchi-Hayakawa, Kazunori Suda, Hiroshi Ishikawa, Yusuke Gondo, Kensuke Shimizu, Takahiro Matsuki, et al. 2016. "Fermented Milk Containing *Lactobacilllus casei* Strain Shirota Preserves the Diversity of the Gut Microbiota and Relieves Abdominal Dysfunction in Healthy Medical Students Exposed to Academic Stress." *Applied and Environmental Microbiology* 82, no. 12 (May): 3649–58. https://doi.org/10.1128/AEM.04134-15.

Kauffmann, T., T. Elvasåshagen, D. Alnæs, N. Zak, P. Ø. Pedersen, L. B. Norbom, S. H. Quraishi, E. Tagliazucchi, H. Laufs, A. Biørnerud, U. F. Malt, et al. 2016. "The Brain Functional Connectome Is Robustly Altered by Lack of Sleep." *Neuroimage* 127 (Feb.): 324–32. https://doi.org/10.1016/j.neuroimage.2015.12.028.

Kavlock, R. J. 1999. "Overview of Endocrine Disruptor Research Activity in the United States." *Chemosphere* 39, no. 8 (Oct.): 1227–36. https://doi.org/10.1016/s0045-6535(99)00190-3.

Kellner, Lindsay. 2017. "The Best Doctor-Approved Supplements to Beat Your Brain Fog." *Mind Body Green.* https://www.mindbodygreen.com/0-29258/the-best-doctorapproved-supplements-to-beat-your-brain-fog.html.

Kennedy, D. O., A. B. Scholey, N. T. Tildesley, E. K. Perry, and K. A. Wesnes. 2002. "Modulation of Mood and Cognitive Performance Following Acute Administration of *Melissa officinalis* (Lemon Balm)." *Pharmacology, Biochemistry, and Behavior* 72, no. 4 (July): 953–64. https://www.ncbi.nlm.nih.gov/pubmed/12062586.

Keville, Kathi, and Mindy Green. 2008. *Aromatherapy: A Complete Guide to the Healing Art.* 2nd ed. New York: Crossing Press.

Khan, N. A., L. B. Raine, E. S. Drollette, M. R. Scudder, A. F. Kramer, and C. H. Hillman. 2015. "Dietary Fiber Is Positively Associated with Cognitive Control Among Prepubertal Children." *Journal of Nutrition* 145, no. 1 (Jan.): 143–49. https://doi.org/10.3945/jn.114.198457.

Kim, H. J. 2007. "Effect of Aromatherapy Massage on Abdominal Fat and Body Image in Post-Menopausal Women." *Taehan Kanho Hakhoe Chi* 37, no. 4 (June): 603–12. https://www.ncbi.nlm.nih.gov/pubmed/17615482.

Kim, Sioh, Hyun-Jae Kim, Jin-Seok Yeo, Sung-Jung Hong, Ji-Min Lee, and Younghoon Jeon. 2011. "The Effect of Lavender Oil on Stress, Bispectral Index Values, and Needle Insertion Pain in Volunteers." *Journal of Alternative and Complementary Medicine* 17, no. 9 (Aug.): 823–26. https://doi.org/10.1089/acm.2010.0644.

Kline, R. M., J. J. Kline, J. Di Palma, and G. J. Barbero. 2001. "Enteric-coated, pH-dependent Peppermint Oil Capsules for the Treatment of Irritable Bowel Syndrome in Children." *Journal of Pediatrics* 138, no. 1 (Jan.): 125–28. https://www.ncbi.nlm.nih.gov/pubmed/11148527.

Konturek, P. C., T. Brzozowski, and S. J. Konturek. 2011. "Stress and the Gut: Pathophysiology, Clinical Consequences, Diagnostic Approach and Treatment Options." *Journal of Physiology and Pharmacology* 62, no. 6 (Dec.): 591–99. https://www.ncbi.nlm.nih.gov/pubmed/22314561.

Koulivand, P. H., M. K. Ghadiri, and A. Gorji. 2013. "Lavender and the Nervous System." *Evidence-Based Complementary and Alternative Medicine* Vol. 2013: 681304. https://doi.org/10.1155/2013/681304.

Kreuder, A. K., D. Scheele, L. Wassermann, M. Wollseifer, B. Stoffel-Wagner, M. R. Lee, J. Hennig, W. Maier, and R. Hurlemann. 2017. "How the Brain Codes Intimacy: The Neurobiological Substrates of Romantic Touch." *Human Brain Mapping* 38, no. 9 (Sept.): 4525–34. https://doi.org/10.1002/hbm.23679.

Lakhan, Shaeen, Heather Sheafer, and Deborah Tepper. 2016. "The Effectiveness of Aromatherapy in Reducing Pain: A Systematic Review and Meta-Analysis." *Pain Research and Treatment* Vol. 2016. https://doi.org/10.1155/2016/8158693.

Lee K. B., E. Cho, and Y. S. Kang. 2014. "Changes in 5-hydroxytryptamine and Cortisol Plasma Levels in Menopausal Women After Inhalation of Clary Sage Oil." *Phytotherapy Research* 28, no. 12 (Dec.): 1897. https://doi.org/10.1002/ptr.5163.

Lehrner, J., G. Marwinski, S. Lehr, P. Johren, and L. Deecke. 2005. "Ambient Odors of Orange and Lavender Reduce Anxiety and Improve Mood in a Dental Office." *Physiology & Behavior* 86, nos. 1–2: 92–95. https://doi.org/10.1016/j.physbeh.2005.06.031.

Leproult, R., and E. Van Cauter. 2010. "Role of Sleep and Sleep Loss in Hormonal Release and Metabolism." *Endocrine Development* 17: 11–21. https://doi.org/10.1159/000262524.

Lewis, M. D. 2016. "Concussions, Traumatic Brain Injury, and the Innovative Use of Omega-3s." *Journal of the American College of Nutrition* 35, no. 5 (July): 469–75. https://doi.org/10.1080/07315724.2016.1150796.

Licznerska, B. E., H. Szaefer, M. Murias, A. Bartoszek, and W. Baer-Dubowska. 2013. "Modulation of CYP19 Expression by Cabbage Juices and Their Active Components: Indole-3-Carbinol and 3,3'-diindolylmethane in Human Breast Epithelial Cell Lines." *European Journal of Nutrition* 52, no. 5 (Aug.): 1483–92. https://doi.org/10.1007/s00394-012-0455-9.

Lillehei, A. S., L. L. Halcón, K. Savik, and R. Reis. 2015. "Effect of Inhaled Lavender and Sleep Hygiene on Self-Reported Sleep Issues: A Randomized Controlled Trial." *Journal of Alternative & Complementary Medicine* 21, no. 7 (July): 430–38. https://doi.org/10.1089.acm.2014.0327.

Lis-Balchin, M. 1997. "Essential Oils and 'Aromatherapy': Their Modern Role in Healing." *Journal of the Royal Society for the Promotion of Health* 177, no. 5: 324–29. http://www.aromaticscience.com/essential-oils-and-aromatherapy-their-modern-role-in-healing-2/.

Liu, J. H., G. H. Chen, H. Z. Yeh, C. K. Huang, and S. K. Poon. 1997. "Enteric-coated Peppermint-Oil Capsules in the Treatment of Irritable Bowel Syndrome: A Prospective, Randomized Trial." *Journal of Gastroenterology* 32, no. 6: 765–68. https://www.ncbi.nlm.nih.gov/pubmed/9430014.

Liu, J., J. E. Burdette, H. Xu, C. Gu, R. B. van Breemen, K. P. Bhat, N. Booth, A. I. Constantinou, J. M. Pezzuto, H. H. Fong, N. R. Farnsworth, and J. L. Bolton. 2001. "Evaluation of Estrogenic Activity of Plant Extracts for the Potential Treatment of Menopausal Symptoms." *Journal of Agricultural and Food Chemistry* 49, no. 5 (May): 2472–79. https://www.ncbi.nlm.nih.gov/pubmed/11368622.

Lobo, V., A. Patil, A. Phatak, and N. Chandra. 2010. "Free Radicals, Antioxidants, and Functional Foods: Impact on Human Health." *Pharmacognosy Reviews* 4, no. 8 (July–Dec.): 118–26. https://doi.org/10.4103.0973-7847.70902.

López, V., B. Nielsen, M. Solas, M. J. Ramirez, and A. K. Jäger. 2017. "Exploring Pharmacological Mechanisms of Lavender (*Lavandula anguistifola*) Essential Oil on Central Nervous System Targets." *Frontiers in Pharmacology* 8 (May): 280. https://doi.org/10.3389/fphar.2017.00280.

Luine, V. N. 2014. "Estradiol and Cognitive Function: Past, Present, and Future." *Hormones and Behavior* 66, no. 4 (Sept.): 602–18. https://doi.org/10.1016/j.yhbeh.2014.08.011.

Lupien, S. J., S. Gaudreau, B. M. Tchiteya, F. Maheu, S. Sharma, N. P. V. Nair, R. L. Hauger, B. S. McEwen, and M. J. Meaney. 1997. "Stress-Induced Declarative Memory Impairment in Healthy Elderly Subjects: Relationship to Cortisol Reactivity." *Journal of Clinical Endocrinology & Metabolism* 82, no. 8 (July): 2070–75. https://doi.org/10.1210/jcem.82.7.4075.

Lytle, Jamie, Catherine Mwatha, and Karen K. Davis. 2014. "Effect of Lavender Aromatherapy on Vital Signs and Perceived Quality of Sleep in the Intermediate Care Unit: A Pilot Study." *American Journal of Critical Care* 23, no. 1 (Jan.): 24–29. https://doi.org/10.4037/ajcc2014958.

Maglich, J. M., M. Kuhn, R. E. Chapin, and M. T. Pletcher. 2014. "More Than Just Hormones: H295R Cells as Predictors of Reproductive Toxicity." *Reproductive Toxicology* 45 (June): 77–86. https://doi.org/10.1016/j.reprotox.2013.12.009.

Mastorakos, G., M. G. Pavlatou, and M. Mizamtsidi. 2006. "The Hypothalamic-Pituitary-Adrenal and the Hypothalamic-Pituitary-Gonadal Axes Interplay." *Pediatric Endocrinology Reviews* 3 Suppl. 1 (Jan.): 172–81. https://www.ncbi.nlm.nih.gov/pubmed/16641855.

Matsumoto, T., Asakura, H., and T. Hayashi. 2013. "Does Lavender Aromatherapy Alleviate Premenstrual Emotional Symptoms?: A Randomized Crossover Trial." *BioPsychoSocial Medicine* 7: 12. https://doi.org/10.1186/1751-0759-7-12.

McAninch, Elizabeth A., and Antonio C. Bianco. 2014. "Thyroid Hormone Signaling in Energy Homeostasis and Energy Metabolism." *Annals of the New York Academy of Sciences* 1311 (Apr.): 77–87. https://doi.org/10.1111/nyas.12374.

McCabe, D., K. Lisy, C. Lockwood, and M. Colbeck. 2017. "The Impact of Essential Fatty Acid, B Vitamins, Vitamin C, Magnesium and Zinc Supplementation on Stress Levels in Women: A Systematic Review." *JBI Database of Systemic Reviews and Implementation Reports* 15, no. 2 (Feb.): 402–53. https://www.ncbi.nlm.nih.gov/pubmed/28178022.

McCraty, R., B. Barrios-Choplin, D. Rozman, M. Atkinson, and A. D. Watkins. 1998. "The Impact of a New Emotional Self-Management Program on Stress, Emotions, Heart Rate Variability, DHEA and Cortisol." *Integrative and Physiological and Behavioral Science* 33, no. 2 (Apr.–June): 151–70. https://www.ncbi.nlm.nih.gov/pubmed/9737736.

Meamarbashi, A. 2014. "Instant Effects of Peppermint Essential Oil on the Physiological Parameters and Exercise Performance." *Avicenna Journal of Phytomedicine* 4, no. 1 (Jan.–Feb.): 72–78. https://www.ncbi.nlm.nih.gov/pmc/articles/PMC4103722/.

Meamarbashi, A., and A. Rajabi. 2013. "The Effects of Peppermint on Exercise Performance." *Journal of the International Society of Sports Nutrition* 10: 15. https://doi.org/10.1186/1550-2783-10-15.

Meeker, J. D. 2012. "Exposure to Environmental Endocrine Disruptors and Child Development." *Archives of Pediatrics and Adolescent Medicine* 166, no. 1: E1–E7. https://doi.org/10.1001/archpediatrics.2012.241.

Meier, U., and A. M. Gressner. 2004. "Endocrine Regulation of Energy Metabolism: Review of Pathobiochemical and Clinical Chemical Aspects of Leptin, Ghrelin, Adiponectin, and Resistin." *Clinical Chemistry* 50, no. 9 (Sept.): 1511–25. https://doi.org/10.1373/clinchem.2004.032482.

Minich, D. M., and J. S. Bland. 2007. "A Review of the Clinical Efficacy and Safety of Cruciferous Vegetable Phytochemicals." *Nutrition Reviews* 65, no. 6, Pt. 1 (June): 259–67. https://www.ncbi.nlm.nih.gov/pubmed/17605302.

Moraes, T. M., H. Kushima, F. C. Moleiro, R. C. Santos, L. R. Rocha, M. O. Marques, W. Vilegas, and C. A. Hiruma-Lima. 2009. "Effects of Limonene and Essential Oil from *Citrus aurantium* on Gastric Mucosa: Role of Prostaglandins and Gastric Mucus Secretion." *Chemico-Biological Interactions* 180, no. 3 (Aug.): 499–505. https://doi.org/10.1016/j.cbi.2009.04.006.

Morhenn, V., L. E. Beavin, and P. J. Zak. 2012. "Massage Increases Oxytocin and Reduces Adrenocorticotropin Hormone in Humans." *Alternative Therapies in Health and Medicine* 18, no. 6 (Nov.–Dec.): 11–18. https://www.ncbi.nlm.nih.gov/pubmed/23251939.

Moss, M., and L. Oliver. 2012. "Plasma 1,8-Cineole Correlates with Cognitive Performance Following Exposure to Rosemary Essential Oil Aroma." *Thera-*

peutic Advances in Psychopharmacology 2, no. 3 (June): 103–13. https://doi
.org/10.1177/2045125312436573.

Moss, M., J. Cook, K. Wesnes, and P. Duckett. 2003. "Aromas of Rosemary and
Lavender Essential Oils Differentially Affect Cognition and Mood in Healthy
Adults." *International Journal of Neuroscience* 113, no. 1 (Jan.): 15–38. https://
www.ncbi.nlm.nih.gov/pubmed/12690999.

Moss, M., S. Hewitt, L. Moss, and K. Wesnes. 2008. "Modulation of Cognitive
Performance and Mood by Aromas of Peppermint and Ylang-Ylang." *International Journal of Neurosciences* 118, no. 1 (Jan.): 59–77. https://www.ncbi
.nlm.nih.gov/pubmed/18041606.

Motomura, N., A. Sakurai, and Y. Yotsuya. 2001. "Reduction of Mental Stress
with Lavender Odorant." *Perceptual and Motor Skills* 93, no. 3: 713–18. https://
doi.org/10.2466/pms.2001.93.3.713.

National Heart, Lung, and Blood Institute—National Institutes of Health. 2017.
"Why Is Sleep Important?" https://www.nhlbi.nih.gov/health/health-topics
/topics/sdd/why.

National Institute on Alcohol Abuse and Alcoholism. 2004. "Alcohol Alert." No.
63. https://pubs.niaaa.nih.gov/publications/aa63/aa63.htm.

National Institute of Environmental Health Sciences. 2017. "Endocrine Disruptors." https://www.niehs.nih.gov/research/supported/exposure/endocrine/
index.cfm.

National Institute of Environmental Health Sciences (NIEHS). 2016. "Perfluorinated Chemicals (PFCs)." https://www.niehs.nih.gov/health/materials/
perflourinated_chemicals_508.pdf.

National Institutes of Health Office of Dietary Supplements. 2017. "Black Cohosh." https://ods.od.nih.gov/factsheets/BlackCohosh-HealthProfessional/.

Nijholt, I., N. Farchi, M. Kye, E. H. Sklan, S. Shoham, B. Verbeure, D. Owen,
B. Hochner, J. Spiess, H. Soreq, and T. Blank. 2004. "Stress-Induced Alternative Splicing of Acetylcholinesterase Results in Enhanced Fear Memory and
Long-Term Potentiation." *Molecular Psychiatry* 9, no 2 (Feb.): 174–83. https://
doi.org/10.1038/sj.mp.4001446.

O'Connor, P. J., M. P. Herring, and A. Carvalho. 2010. "Mental Health Benefits
of Strength Training in Adults." *American Journal of Lifestyle Medicine* 5:
377–96. http://journals.sagepub.com/doi/abs/10.1177/1559827610368771.

Ou, M.C., T. F. Hsu, A. C. Lai, Y. T. Lin, and C. C. Lin. 2012. "Pain Relief Assessment by Aromatic Essential Oil Massage on Outpatients with Primary
Dysmenorrhea: A Randomized, Double-Blind Clinical Trial." *Journal of
Obstetrics and Gynaecology Research* 38, no. 5 (May): 817–22. https://doi
.org/10.1111/j.1447-0756.2011.01802.x.

Ovadje, P., S. Ammar, J. A. Guerrero, J. T. Arnason, and S. Pandey. 2016. "Dandelion Root Extract Affects Colorectal Cancer Proliferation and Survival
Through the Activation of Multiple Death Signaling Pathways." *Oncotarget*
7, no. 45 (Nov.): 73080–100. https://doi.org/10.18632/oncotarget.11485.

Ozen, S. and S. Darcan. 2011. "Effects of Environmental Endocrine Disruptors on Pubertal Development." *Journal of Clinical Residential Pediatric Endocrinology* 3, no. 1 (Mar.): 1–6. https://doi.org/10.4274/jcrpe.v3i1.01.

Pan-Vazquez, A., N. Rye, M. Ameri, B. McSparron, G. Smallwood, J. Bickerdyke, A. Rathbone, F. Dajas-Bailador, and M. Toledo-Rodriguez. 2015. "Impact of Voluntary Exercise and Housing Conditions on Hippocampal Glucocorticoid Receptor, miR-124 and Anxiety." *Molecular Brain* 8 (July): 40. https://doi.org/10.1186/s13041-015-0128-8.

Pappas, Dr. Robert. 2017. "Essential Oil Myths." *Essential Oil University.* http://essentialoils.org/news/eo_myths.

Patki, G., L. Li, F. Allam, N. Solanki, A. T. Dao, K. Alkadhi, and S. Salim. 2014. "Moderate Treadmill Exercise Rescues Anxiety and Depression-Like Behavior as Well as Memory Impairment in a Rat Model of Posttraumatic Stress Disorder." *Physiology & Behavior* 130 (May): 47–53. https://doi.org/ 10.1016/j.physbeh.2014.03.016.

Pemberton, E., and P. G. Turpin. 2008. "The Effect of Essential Oils on Work-Related Stress in Intensive Care Unit Nurses." *Holistic Nursing Practice* 22, no. 2: 97–102. https://doi.org/10.1097/01.hnp.0000312658.13890.28.

Peretz, Jackye, Lisa Vrooman, William A. Ricke, Patricia A. Hunt, Shelley Ehrlich, Russ Hauser, Vasantha Padmanabhan, Hugh S. Taylor, Shanna H. Swan, Catherine A. VandeVoort, et al. 2014. "Bisphenol A and Reproductive Health: Update of Experimental and Human Evidence, 2007–2013." *Environmental Health Perspectives* 122, no. 8 (Aug.): 775–86. https://doi.org/10.1289/ehp.1307728.

Perry, N., and E. Perry. 2006. "Aromatherapy in the Management of Psychiatric Disorders: Clinical and Neuropharmacological Perspectives." *CNS Drugs* 20, no. 4: 257–80. https://www.ncbi.nlm.nih.gov/pubmed/16599645.

Perry, N. S., C. Bollen, E. K. Perry, and C. Ballard. 2003. "Salvia for Dementia Therapy: Review of Pharmacological Activity and Pilot Tolerability Clinical Trial." *Pharmacology, Biochemistry, & Behavior* 75, no. 3 (June): 651–59. https://www.ncbi.nlm.nih.gov/pubmed/12895683.

Pert, Candace B. 1999. *Molecules of Emotion: The Science Behind Mind-Body Medicine.* New York: Simon & Schuster.

Picciotto, M., M. J. Higley, and Y. S. Mineur. 2012. "Acetylcholine as a Neuromodulator: Cholinergic Signaling Shapes Nervous System Function and Behavior." *Neuron* 76, no. 1 (Oct.): 116–29. https://doi.org/10.1016/j.neuron.2012.08.036.

Pilkington, K., G. Kirkwood, H. Rampes, and J. Richardson. 2005. "Yoga for Depression: The Research Evidence." *Journal of Affective Disorders* 89, nos. 1–3 (Dec.): 13–24. https://doi.org/10.1016/j.jad.2005.08.013.

Pizzorno, J. 2014. "Toxins from the Gut." *Integrative Medicine: A Clinician's Journal* 13, no. 6 (Dec.): 8–11. https://www.ncbi.nlm.nih.gov/pmc/articles/PMC4566437/.

Plotsky, P. M., M. J. Owens, and C. B. Nemeroff. 1998. "Psychoneuroendocrinology of Depression. Hypothalamic-Pituitary-Adrenal Axis." *Psychiatric Clin-*

ics of North America 21, no. 2 (June): 293–307. https://www.ncbi.nlm.nih
.gov/pubmed/9670227.

Price, S., and L. Price. 2012. *Aromatherapy for Health Professionals*. London: Churchill Livingstone Elsevier.

Pu, Hongjian, Xiaoyan Jiang, Zhihuo Wei, Dandan Hong, Sulaiman Hassan, Wenting Zhang, Jialin Liu, Hengxing Meng, Yejie Shi, Ling Chen, et al. 2017. "Repetitive and Prolonged Omega-3 Fatty Acid Treatment After Traumatic Brain Injury Enhances Long-Term Tissue Restoration and Cognitive Recovery." *Cell Transplant* 26, no. 4 (Apr.): 555–69. https://doi.org/10.3727/096368916X693842.

Purcheon, Nerys, and Lora Cantele. 2014. *The Complete Aromatherapy & Essential Oils Handbook for Everyday Wellness*. Toronto: Robert Rose.

Radley, J. J., R. M. Anderson, B. A. Hamilton, J. A. Alcock, and S. A. Romig-Martin. 2013. "Chronic Stress-Induced Alterations of Dendritic Spine Subtypes Predict Functional Decrements in an Hypothalamo-Pituitary-Adrenal-Inhibitory Prefrontal Circuit." *Journal of Neurosciences* 33, no. 36 (Sept.): 14379–91. https://doi.org/10.1523/jneurosci.0287-13.2013.

Rajoria, Shilpi, Robert Suriano, Perminder Singh Parmar, Yshan Lisa Wilson, Uchechukwu Megwalu, Augustine Moscatello, H. Leon Bradlow, Daniel W. Sepkovic, et al. 2011. "3,3'-Diindolylmethane Modulates Estrogen Metabolism in Patients with Thyroid Proliferative Disease: A Pilot Study." *Thyroid* 21, no. 3 (Mar.): 299–304. https://doi.org/10.1089/thy.2010.0245.

Ranabir, S., and K. Reetu. 2011. "Stress and Hormones." *Indian Journal of Endocrinology and Metabolism* 15, no. 1 (Jan.–Mar.): 18–22. https://doi.org/10.4103/.2230-8210.77573.

Rapaport, Mark H., Pamela Schettler, and Catherine Bresee. 2012. "A Preliminary Study of the Effects of Repeated Massage on Hypothalamic-Pituitary-Adrenal and Immune Function in Healthy Individuals: A Study of Mechanisms of Action and Dosage." *Journal of Alternative and Complementary Medicine* 18, no. 8 (Aug.): 789–97. doi: 10.1089/acm.2011.0071.

Reichling, J., P. Schnitzler, U. Suschke, and R. Saller. 2009. "Essential Oils of Aromatic Plants with Antibacterial, Antifungal, Antiviral, and Cytotoxic Properties—An Overview." *Forschende Komplementarmedizen* 16, no. 2 (Apr.): 79–90. https://doi.org/10.1159/000207196.

Reis, F. G., R. H. Marques, C. M. Starling, R. Almeida-Reis, R. P. Vieira, C. T. Cabido, L. F. Silva, T. Lanças, M. Dolhnikoff, M. A. Martins, et al. 2012. "Stress Amplifies Lung Tissue Mechanics, Inflammation and Oxidative Stress Induced by Chronic Inflammation." *Experimental Lung Research* 38, no. 7 (Sept.): 344–54. https://doi.org/10.3109/01902148.2012.704484.

Rice, K. M., E. M. Walker, Jr., M. Wu, C. Gillette, and E. R. Blough. 2014. "Environmental Mercury and Its Toxic Effects." *Journal of Preventive Medicine & Public Health* 47, no. 2 (Mar.): 74–93. https://doi.org/10.3961/jpmph.2014.47.2.74.

RMS Beauty. 2017. *Beauty Truth*. http://beautytruth.com.

Rodriguez, Damian, DHSc, MS. 2017. "Emotional Aromatherapy—Science Meets Chemistry." *DoTERRA Science*. https://www.doterra.com/US/en/blog/

science-safety-physiology-emotional-aromatherapy-psychology-meets
-chemistry.

Rombolà, L., L. Tridico, D. Scuteri, T. Sakurada, S. Sakurada, H. Mizoguchi, P. Avato, M. T. Corasaniti, G. Bagetta., and L. A. Morrone. 2017. "Bergamot Essential Oil Attenuates Anxiety-Like Behaviour in Rats." *Molecules* 22, no. 4 (Apr.): 614. https://doi.org/10.3390/molecules22040614.

Romm, Aviva. 2017. *The Adrenal Thyroid Revolution: A Proven 4-Week Program to Rescue Your Metabolism, Hormones, Mind & Mood.* New York: HarperOne.

Roussouw, J. E., G. L. Anderson, R. L Prentice, A. Z. La Croix, C. Kooperberg, M. L. Stefanick, R. D. Jackson, S. A. Beresford, B. V. Howard, K. C. Johnson, J. M. Kotchen, J. Ockene, and Writing Group for the Women's Health Initiative. 2002. "Risks and Benefits of Estrogen Plus Progestin in Healthy Postmenopausal Women: Principal Results from the Women's Health Initiative Randomized Controlled Trial." *JAMA* 288, no. 3 (July): 321–33. https://www.ncbi.nlm.nih.gov/pubmed/12117397.

Saanijoki, Tina, Lauri Tuominen, Jetro J. Tuular, Lauri Nummenmaa, Eveliina Arponen, Kari Kalliokoski, and Jussi Hirvonen. 2017. "Opioid Release After High-Intensity Interval Training in Healthy Human Subjects." *Neuropsychopharmacology* 43 (July): 246–54. https://doi.org/10.1038/npp.2017.148.

Sabogal-Guáqueta, A. M., E. Osorio, and G. P. Cardona-Gómez. 2016. "Linalool Reverses Neuropathological and Behavioral Impairments in Old Triple Transgenic Alzheimer's Mice." *Neuropharmacology* 102 (Mar.): 111–20. https://doi.org/10.1016/j.neuropharm.2015.11.002.

Safer Chemicals, Healthy Families. 2017. "Perfluorinated Compounds (PFCs)." http://saferchemicals.org/chemicals/pfcs/.

Salthouse, T. A. 2010. "Selective Review of Cognitive Aging." *Journal of the International Neuropsychological Society* 16, no. 5 (Sept.): 754–60. https://doi.org/10.1017/S1355617710000706.

Sanderson, H., R. A Brain, D. J. Johnson, C. J. Wilson, and K. R. Solomon. 2004. "Toxicity Classification and Evaluation of Four Pharmaceuticals Classes: Antibiotics, Antineoplastics, Cardiovascular, and Sex Hormones." *Toxicology* 203, nos. 1–3 (Oct.): 27–40. https://doi.org/10.1016/j.tox.2004.05.015.

Santoro, N., G. D. Braunstein, C. L. Butts, K. A. Martin, M. McDermott, and J. V. Pinkerton. 2016. "Compounded Bioidentical Hormones in Endocrinology Practice: An Endocrine Society Scientific Statement." *Journal of Clinical Endocrinology & Metabolism* 101, no. 4 (Apr.): 1318–43. https://doi.org/10.1210/jc.2016-1271.

Sayorwan, W., N. Ruangrungski, T. Piriyapunyporn, T. Hongratanaworakit, N. Kotchabhakdi, and V. Siripornpanich. 2013. "Effects of Inhaled Rosemary Oil on Subjective Feelings and Activities of the Nervous System." *Scientia Pharmaceutica* 81, no. 2 (Apr.–June): 531–42. https://doi.org/10.3797/scipharm.1209-05.

Saxena, Ram Chandra, Rakesh Singh, Parveen Kumar, Mahenra P. Singh Negi, Vinod S. Saxena, Periasamy Geetharani, Joseph Joshua Allan, and Kudiganti Venkateshwarlu. 2012. "Efficacy of an Extract of *Ocimumm tenuiflorum* in the Management of General Stress: A Double-Blind, Placebo-Controlled Study." *Evidence-Based Complementary Alternative Medicine* Vol. 2012 (Oct.): 894509. https://doi.org/10.1155/2012/894509.

Schmitz, K. H., P. J. Hannan, S. D. Stovitz, C. J. Bryan, M. Warren, and M. D. Jensen. 2007. "Strength Training and Adiposity in Premenopausal Women: Strong, Healthy, and Empowered Study." *American Journal of Clinical Nutrition* 86, no. 3 (Sept.): 566–72. https://www.ncbi.nlm.nih.gov/pubmed/17823418.

Schnaubelt, Dr. Kurt. 2011. *The Healing Intelligence of Essential Oils: The Science of Advanced Aromatherapy.* Rochester, VT: Healing Arts Press.

Schwabe, L., M. Joëls, B. Roozendaal, O. T. Wolf, and M. S. Oitzl. 2012. "Stress Effects on Memory: An Update and Integration." *Neuroscience & Biobehavioral Reviews* 36, no. 7 (Aug.): 1740–49. https://doi.org/10.1016/j.neubiorev.2011.07.002.

Seol, G. H., H. S. Shim, P. J. Kim, H. K. Moon, K. H. Lee, I. Shim, S. H. Suh, and S. S. Min. 2010. "Antidepressant-Like Effect of *Salvia sclarea* Is Explained by Modulation of Dopamine Activities in Rats." *Journal of Ethnopharmacology* 130, no. 1 (July): 187–90. https://doi.org/10.1016/j.jep.2010.04.035.

Shen, Y. H., and R. Nahas. 2009. "Complementary and Alternative Medicine for Treatment of Irritable Bowel Syndrome." *Canadian Family Physician* 55, no. 2 (Feb.): 143–48. https://www.ncbi.nlm.nih.gov/pubmed/19221071.

Shinohara, K., H. Doi, C. Kumagai, E. Sawano, and W. Tarumi. 2017. "Effects of Essential Oil Exposure on Salivary Estrogen Concentration in Perimenopausal Women." *Neuro Endocrinology Letters* 37, no. 8 (Jan.): 567–72. https://www.ncbi.nlm.nih.gov/pubmed/?term=geranium+menopause.

Shumaker, Sally A., Claudine Legault, Stephen R. Rapp, Leon Thal, Robert B. Wallace, Judith K. Ockene, Susan L. Hendrix, Beverly N. Jones III, Annlouise R. Assaf, Rebecca D. Jackson, et al. 2003. "Estrogen Plus Progestin and the Incidence of Dementia and Mild Cognitive Impairment in Postmenopausal Women: The Women's Health Initiative Memory Study, a Randomized Controlled Trial." *JAMA* 289, no. 20 (May): 2651–62. https://doi.org/10.1001/jama.289.20.2651.

Sienkiewicz, M., M. Lysakowska, J. Ciećwierz, P. Denys, and E. Kowalczyk. 2011. "Antibacterial Activity of Thyme and Lavender Essential Oils." *Medicinal Chemistry* 7, no. 6 (Nov.): 674–89. https://www.ncbi.nlm.nih.gov/pubmed/22313307.

Sigurdsson, H. H., J. Kirsch, and C. M. Lehr. 2013. "Mucus as a Barrier to Lipophilic Drugs." *International Journal of Pharmaceutics* 453, no. 1 (Aug.): 56–64. https://doi.org/10.1016/j.ijpharm.2013.05.040.

Singh, Narendra, Mohit Bhalla, Prashanti de Jager, and Marilena Gilca. 2011. "An Overview on Ashwagandha: A Rasayana (Rejuvenator) of Ayurveda." *African Journal of Traditional, Complementary and Alternative Medicines* 8, no. 5, Suppl. (July): 208–13. https://doi.org/10.4314/ajtcam.v8i5S.9.

Sinha, R. 2017. "Role of Addiction and Stress Neurobiology on Food Intake and Obesity." *Biological Psychology,* May. https://doi.org/10.1016/j.biopsycho.2017.05.001.

Sinha, R., and A. M. Jastreboff. 2013. "Stress as a Common Risk Factor for Obesity and Addiction." *Biological Psychiatry* 73, no. 9 (May): 827–35. https://doi.org/10.1016/j.biopsych.2013.01.032.

Snyder, Mariza. 2017. *Smart Mom's Guide to Essential Oils.* Berkeley, CA: Ulysses Press.

Snyder, Mariza. 2017. "Top 5 Detoxing Essential Oils to Reduce Toxic Load." https://www.drmariza.com/top-detoxing-essential-oils-to-reduce-toxic-load/.

Snyder, Mariza, and Lauren Clum. 2014. *Water Infusions: Refreshing, Detoxifying and Healthy Recipes for Your Home Infuser.* Berkeley, CA: Ulysses Press.

Soreq, H. 2015. "Checks and Balances on Cholinergic Signaling in Brain and Body Function." *Trends in Neuroscience* 38, no. 7 (July): 448–58. https://doi.org/10.1016/j.tins.2015.05.007.

Soto-Vásquez, Manilu, and Paul Alan Arkin Alvarado-García. 2017. "Aromatherapy with Two Essential Oils from *Satureja* Genre and Mindfulness Meditation to Reduce Anxiety in Humans." *Journal of Traditional and Complementary Medicine* 7, no. 1 (Jan.): 121–25. https://doi.org/10.1016/j.jtcme.2016.06.003.

Speciale, A., J. Chirafisi, A. Jaija, and F. Cimino. 2011. "Nutritional Antioxidants and Adaptive Cell Responses: An Update." *Current Molecular Medicine* 11, no. 9 (Dec.): 770–89. https://www.ncbi.nlm.nih.gov/pubmed/21999148.

Steiner, M., E. Dunn, and L. Born. 2003. "Hormones and Mood: From Menarche to Menopause and Beyond." *Journal of Affective Disorders* 74, no. 1 (Mar.): 67–83. https://doi.org/10.1016/S0165-0327(02)00432-9.

Stengel, A., and Y. Tache. 2009. "Neuroendocrine Control of the Gut During Stress: Corticotropin-Releasing Factor Signaling Pathways in the Spotlight." *Annual Review of Physiology* 71: 219–39. https://doi.org/10.1146/annurev.physiol.010908.163221.

Stonehouse, W., C. A. Conion, J. Podd, S. R. Hill, A. M. Minihane, C. Haskell, and D. Kennedy. 2013. "DHA Supplementation Improved Both Memory and Reaction Time in Healthy Young Adults: A Randomized Controlled Trial." *American Journal of Clinical Nutrition* 97, no. 5 (May): 1134–43. https://doi.org/10.3945/ajcn.112.053371.

Sumedha, M. J. 2008. "The Sick Building Syndrome." *Indian Journal of Occupational & Environmental Medicine* 12, no. 2 (Aug.): 61–64. https://doi.org/10.4103/0019-5278.43262.

Taheri, Shahrad, Ling Lin, Diane Austin, Terry Young, and Emmanuel Mignot. 2004. "Short Sleep Duration Is Associated with Reduced Leptin, Elevated Ghrelin, and Increased Body Mass Index." *PLoS Med* 1, no. 3 (Dec.): e62. https://doi.org/10.1371/journal.pmed.0010062.

Takaya, J., H. Higashino, and Y. Kobayashi. 2004. "Intracellular Magnesium and Insulin Resistance." *Magnesium Research* 17, no. 2 (June): 126–36. https://www.ncbi.nlm.nih.gov/pubmed/15319146.

Tan, Loh Teng Hern, Learn Han Lee, Wai Fong Yin, Chim Kei Chan, Habsah Abdul Kadir, Kok Gan Chan, and Bey Hing Goh. 2015. "Traditional Uses, Phytochemistry, and Bioactivities of *Cananga odorata* (Ylang-Ylang)." *Evidence-*

Based Complementary & Alternative Medicine Vol. 2015: 896314. https://doi
.org/10.1155/2015/896314.

Tendzegolskis, Z., A. Viru, and E. Orlova. 1991. "Exercise-Induced Changes of
Endorphin Contents in Hypothalamus, Hypophysis, Adrenals and Blood
Plasma." *International Journal of Sports Medicine* 12, no. 5 (Oct.): 495–97.
https://doi.org/10.1055/s-2007-1024721.

Tesch, B. J. 2002. "Herbs Commonly Used by Women: An Evidence-Based Review." *Disease-a-Month* 48, no. 10 (Oct.): 671–96. https://www.ncbi.nlm.nih
.gov/pubmed/12562054.

Thaiss, C. A., D. Zeevi, M. Levy, G. Zilberman-Schapira, J. Suez, A. C. Tengeier,
L. Abramson, M. N. Katz, T. Korem, N. Zimora, Y. Kuperman, I. Biton, et
al. 2014. "Transkingdom Control of Microbiota Diurnal Oscillations Promotes Metabolic Homeostasis." *Cell* 159, no. 3 (Oct.): 514–29. https://doi
.org/10.1016/j.cell.2014.09.048.

Thoma, Myriam V., Roberta La Marca, Rebecca Brönnimann, Linda Finkel,
Ulrike Ehlert, and Urs M. Nater. 2013. "The Effect of Music on the Human
Stress Response." *PLos One* 8, no. 8 (Aug.): e70156. https://doi.org/10.1371/
journal.pone.0070156.

Thomas, H. N., M. Hamm, R. Hess, and R. C. Thurston. 2017. "Changes in Sexual
Function Among Midlife Women: 'I'm Older . . . and I'm Wiser.'" *Menopause*,
October. https://doi.org/10.1097/GME.0000000000000988.

Tildesley, N. T., D. O. Kennedy, E. K. Perry, C. G. Ballard, S. Saveley, K. A.
Wesnes, and A. B. Scholey. 2003. "*Salvia lavandulaefolia* (Spanish Sage)
Enhances Memory in Healthy Young Volunteers." *Pharmacology, Biochemistry, & Behavior* 75, no. 3 (June): 669–74. https://www.ncbi.nlm.nih.gov/
pubmed/12895685.

TIME Health. 2014. "12 Unexpected Things That Mess with Your Memory."
Time. (Aug. 14). http://time.com/3195795/12-unexpected-things-that-mess
-with-your-memory/.

Toda, M., and K. Morimoto. 2008. "Effect of Lavender Aroma on Salivary En-
docrinological Stress Markers." *Archives of Oral Biology* 53, no. 10: 964–68.
https://doi.org/10.1016/j.archoralbio.2008.04.002.

Total Wellness Publishing. 2015. *The Essential Life.* 2nd ed. Jackson, WY: Total
Wellness.

Tseng, H. C., J. H. Grendell, and S. S. Rothman. 1984. "Regulation of Digestion.
II. Effects of Insulin and Glucagon on Pancreatic Secretion." *American Journal of Physiology* 246, no. 4 Pt. 1 (Apr.): G451–56. https://doi.org/10.1152/
ajpgi.1984.246.4.G451.

Unuvar, T., and A. Buyukgebiz. 2012. "Fetal and Neonatal Endocrine Disruptors." *Journal of Clinical Research in Pediatric Endocrinology* 4, no. 2 (June):
51–60. https://doi.org/10.4274/Jcrpe.569.

U.S. Electronic Code of Federal Regulations (e-CFR). 2017. "Substances Generally Recognized as Safe—182.20 Essential Oils, Oleoresins (Solvent-Free),
and Natural Extractives (Including Distillates)." https://www.ecfr.gov/
cgi-bin/text-idx?rgn=div5&node=21:3.0.1.1.13#se21.3.182_120.

Van den Beld, Annewieke, Theo J. Visser, Richard A. Feelders, Diederick E. Grobbee, and Steven W. J. Lamberts. 2005. "Thyroid Hormone Concentrations, Disease, Physical Function, and Mortality in Elderly Men." *Journal of Clinical Endocrinology and Metabolism* 90, no. 12 (Dec.): 6403–409. https://doi.org/10.1210/jc.2005-0872.

Van Die, M. D., H. G. Burger, H. J. Teede, and K. M. Bone. 2013. "*Vitex agnus-castus* Extracts for Female Reproductive Disorders: A Systematic Review of Clinical Trials." *Planta Medica* 79, no. 7 (May): 562–75. https://doi.org/10.1055/s-0032-1327831.

Vgontzas, A. N., E. O. Bixler, H. M. Lin, P. Prolo, G. Mastorakos, A. Vela-Bueno, A. Kales, and G. P. Chrousos. 2001. "Chronic Insomnia Is Associated with Nyctohemeral Activation of the Hypothalamic-Pituitary-Adrenal Axis: Clinical Implications." *Journal of Clinical Endocrinology & Metabolism* 86, no. 8 (Aug.): 3787–94. https://doi.org/10.1210/jcem.86.8.7778.

Voynow, J. A., and B. K. Rubin. 2009. "Mucins, Mucus, and Sputum." *Chest* 135, no. 2 (Feb.): 505–12. https://doi.org/10/1378/chest.08-0412.

Wagner, M., and J. Oehlmann. 2009. "Endocrine Disruptors in Bottled Mineral Water: Total Estrogenic Burden and Migration from Plastic Bottles." *Environmental Science and Pollution Research International* 16, no. 3 (May): 278–86. https://doi.org/10.1007/s11356-009-0107-7.

Walker, A. F., M. C. De Souza, M. F. Vickers, S. Abeyasekera, M. L. Collins, and L. A. Trinca. 1998. "Magnesium Supplementation Alleviates Premenstrual Symptoms of Fluid Retention." *Journal of Women's Health* 7, no. 9 (Nov.): 1157–64. https://www.ncbi.nlm.nih.gov/pubmed/9861593.

Washington University in St. Louis. 2015. "Earlier Menopause Linked to Everyday Chemical Exposures." *ScienceDaily.* https://www.sciencedaily.com/releases/2015/01/150128141417.htm.

Watanabe, E., K. Kuchta, M. Kimura, H. W. Rauwald, T. Kamei, and J. Imanishi. 2015. "Effects of Bergamot (*Citrus bergamia* (Risso) Wright & Arn.) Essential Oil Aromatherapy on Mood States, Parasympathetic Nervous System Activity, and Salivary Cortisol Levels in 41 Healthy Females." *Forschende Komplementärmedizin* 22, no. 1: 43–49. https://doi.org/10.1159/000380989.

Weaver, Libby. 2016. *Accidentally Overweight.* New York: Hay House.

Weil, E. 2012. "Puberty Before Age 10: A New Normal?" *New York Times* (March 30). http://www.nytimes.com/2012/04/01/magazine/puberty-before-age-10-a-new-normal.html?_r=2.

Weinberg, Lisa, Anita Hasni, Minoru Shinhara, and Audrey Duarte. 2014. "A Single Bout of Resistance Exercise Can Enhance Episodic Memory Performance." *Acta Psychologica* 153 (Nov.): 13–19. https://doi.org/10.1016/j.actpsy.2014.06.011.

Whedon, James M., Anupama KizhakkeVeettil, Nancy A. Rugo, and Kelly A. Kieffer. 2017. "Bioidentical Estrogen for Menopausal Depressive Symptoms: A Systematic Review and Meta-Analysis." *Journal of Women's Health* (*Larchmt*) 26, no. 1 (Jan.): 18–28. https://doi.org/10.1089/jwh.2015.5628.

Women's Voices for the Earth (WVE). 2017. "Why a Woman's Organization— The Impact of Toxic Chemicals on Women's Health." https://www.womens voices.org/about/why-a-womens-organization.

World Health Organization (WHO). 2017. "Arsenic Factsheet." http://www.who .int/mediacentre/factsheets/fs372/en/.

World Health Organization (WHO). 2017. "Mercury and Health Fact Sheet." http://www.who.int/mediacentre/factsheets/fs361/en/.

World Health Organization (WHO). 2009. "Tobacco." http://www.who.int/ nmh/publications/fact_sheet_tobacco_en.pdf.

Wu, Yani, Yinan Zhang, Guoxiang Xie, Xiaolan Pan, Tianlu Chen, Yixue Hu, Yumin Liu, Yi Chi, Lei Yao, and Wei Jia. 2012. "The Metabolic Responses to Aerial Diffusion of Essential Oils." *PLoSOne* 7, no. 9 (Sept.): e44830. https:// doi.org/10.1371/journal.pone.0044830.

Yang, Dicheng, Jing Li, Zhongxiang Yan, and Xu Liu. 2013. "Effect of Hormone Replacement Therapy on Cardiovascular Outcomes: A Meta-Analysis of Randomized Controlled Trials." *PLoSOne* 8, no. 5 (May): e62329. https://doi .org/10.1371/journal.pone.0062329.

Youdim, K. A., and S. G. Deans. 2000. "Effect of Thyme Oil and Thymol Dietary Supplementation on the Antioxidant Status and Fatty Acid Composition of the Aging Rat Brain." *British Journal of Nutrition* 83, no. 1 (Jan.): 87–93. https://www.ncbi.nlm.nih.gov/pubmed/10703468.

Young, S. N. 2007. "How to Increase Serotonin in the Human Brain Without Drugs." *Journal of Psychiatry & Neuroscience* 32, no. 6 (Nov.): 394–99. https:// www.ncbi.nlm.nih.gov/pmc/articles/PMC2077351/.

Zava, D. R., Dollbaum, C. M., and Blen, M. 1998. "Estrogen and Progestin Bioactivity of Foods, Herbs, and Spices." *Proceedings of the Society for Experimental Biology and Medicine* 217, no. 3 (Mar): 369–78. https://www.ncbi.nlm.nih .gov/pubmed/9492350.

Zeligs, M. A., and A. S. Connelly. 2000. *All About DIM.* New York: Penguin.

Zenko, Z., P. Ekkekakis, and D. Ariely. 2016. "Can You Have Your Vigorous Exercise and Enjoy It Too? Ramping Intensity Down Increases Postexercise, Remembered, and Forecasted Pleasure." *Journal of Sport & Exercise Psychology* 38, no. 2 (Apr.): 149–59. https://doi.org/10.1123/jsep.2015-0286.

Zipursky, Rachel T., Marcella Calfon Press, Preethi Srikanthan, Jeff Gornbein, Robyn McClelland, Karol Watson, and Tamara B. Horwich. 2017. "Relation of Stress Hormones (Urinary Catecholamines/Cortisol) to Coronary Artery Calcium in Men Versus Women (from the Multi-Ethnic Study of Atherosclerosis [MESA])." *American Journal of Cardiology* 119, no. 12 (June): 1963–71. https://doi.org/10.1016/j.amjcard.2017.03.025.

Zouhal, H., S. Lemoine-Morel, M. E. Mathieu, G. A. Casazza, and G. Jabbour. 2013. "Catecholamines and Obesity: Effects of Exercise and Training." *Sports Medicine* 43, no. 7 (July): 591–600. https://doi.org/10.1007/ s40279-013-0039-8.

Acknowledgments

Thank You!

I want to thank the following people for supporting me in creating this book and getting it out into the world to serve beautiful, remarkable women.

Alex Dunks, my incredible husband—for supporting me during those long nights testing recipes and writing the book. You are amazing and the best partner I could have on this incredible journey.

My beautiful mom, Jody DeLeone, for allowing me to share your journey and for inspiring me to reach for the stars and to never give up!

My grandmothers, Rachel Anguiano and Sharon Snyder, for your unwavering support. Each of you have shaped me to be the woman I am today.

Ellena, Nicole, Kristen, Amanda, Emily, and the rest of my rockstar team behind the scenes—making our mission possible and allowing me to stay focused on my passion projects. I am so grateful for your support and dedication every day.

My amazing community of essential oil rock stars that I get to work with every day who change lives by sharing and educating about the benefits of self care and essential oils. You are making a huge difference in this world, one drop at a time.

Jolene Brighten—for your amazing friendship as we navigate this book journey together. J. J. Virgin—for being a powerful inspiration, mentor, and friend. Magdalena Wszelaki—for giving me real talk advice along the way. Robyn Openshaw—for supporting me since I began this journey many years ago. Bridgit Danner—for being my light and our countless weekly phone calls. Karl Krummenacher—for giving me clarity and keeping me on track with the bigger picture.

Amanda Olsen—for being my cheerleader and always knowing what to say. Candace Romero—for having my back since I was twenty-two years old and giving me great insight on what women want out of this book. Tony Youn—for believing in me and having my back! Cynthia Snyder—for being the best sister.

To all of my fellow wellness rock stars: Zia Nix, Brianne Hovey, Bree Argetsinger, Amy Medling, Nicole Willis, Izabella and Michael Wentz, Trevor Cates, Steph Gaudreau, Nicole Jardim, Garbielle Lyon, Lauren Noel, Erin Nielson, Melissa Kathryn, Dave Asprey, Katie Wells, Teri Cochrane, Emily Fletcher, Alex Carrasco, Alexandra Jamieson, Ann Shippy, Kevin and Annmarie Gianni, Anna Cabeca, Melissa Esguerra, Christiana Maia, Cynthia Pasquela, Elisa Song, Summer Bock, Jerry Bailey, Joan Rosenberg, Alan and Kirin Christianson, Kellyann Petrucci, Mallory Leone, Jessica Drummond, Amy Myers, Maru Davila, Nat Kringoudis, Robyn Benson, Tricia Nelson, Trudy Scott, Will Cole, Lara Adler, and Vincent Pedre—together we are changing the world!

My incredible publishing team—Wendy Sherman, thank you for being the best literary agent and having faith in me every step of the way. Your unwavering support and commitment are awe-inspiring. Karen Moline and Erin Hubbard for helping me to create this book and making it approachable for my readers. Your guidance from start to finish was invaluable.

Anna Z. Bohbot for being my fellow collaborator in all of my books and for creating incredible recipes. The wonderful team at Harmony Books for partnering with me to create this book—Alyse Diamond, Christina Foxley, Danielle Curtis, Tammy Blake, Connie Capone, and all of the rock stars in the copyediting department.

To my readers—I am so grateful to you for allowing me to be a part of your awesome healing journey. You are the reason I wrote this book.